THE JONATHAN ATKINS

Develop the
Power to
Heal

A dedicated healer, Pat Butler successfully treated thousands of patients in the UK for over 20 years. He was a member of six healing organisations and Chairman of the Suffolk Healers Association in the UK, for whom he trained many new healers. As well as publishing numerous articles, he was interviewed for both TV and radio and was a prominent advocate of developing one's own healing abilities.

Develop the Power to Heal

Patrick Butler

quantum

LONDON • NEW YORK • TORONTO • SYDNEY

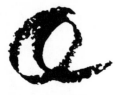

quantum

An imprint of W. Foulsham & Co. Ltd
The Publishing House, Bennetts Close,
Cippenham, Berkshire, SL1 5AP, England

ISBN 0-572-02516-5

Printed in Great Britain by St Edmundsbury Press, Bury St Edmunds, Suffolk

Contents

Dedicated to the memory of Gordon Turner, a great healer

Foreword

Reading this book has reminded me of many of the exercises which helped me in my own personal development and there will be many healers who have had experiences similar to Patrick Butler's. For these reasons, this book is of particular value since it offers an excellent and well-proven series of exercises for the beginner. Do not underestimate the simplicity of the programme. If these exercises are completed over a period of time, then progress will be made in a safe and secure way.

The decade of the 1980s saw a dramatic increase in the public awareness of all aspects of complementary medicine. Public opinion polls have shown that 80 per cent of those surveyed would like to see complementary medicine embraced by mainstream medicine. Other surveys have shown that 75 per cent of all referrals to complementary practitioners in the UK come from satisfied clients.

The media have also played their part in stimulating interest in all types of healing by means of articles which describe the various treatments, and these bring a flood of enquiries from those who have not been cured by other means.

Many doctors, nurses and other health professionals now recognise that all the healing arts have a part to play in the future of health care. The overall consciousness has changed and now, instead of viewing complementary therapies as 'alternative' to the NHS, most people see the need to provide the appropriate treatment to help the patient back to full health and strength. Complementary medicine is concerned with the body, mind, emotions and vitality or spirit of the individual, and consequently all practitioners can play their part.

In short, complementary medicine is holism in practice.

At the root of all health care is the natural response of the individual to repair the body and remain healthy. The natural healing mechanism and the way in which patients can be encouraged to regain their health can take many forms and it must be for individuals to make their own choice. The enquirer may find it is useful to experience a number of different approaches to healing in order to find the one that is most comfortable. It is well to remember that as we progress along the path of learning, we bring our own special contribution to the work and our attitudes may change. This is to be expected.

To be able to help and encourage the healing process in those who are suffering is a most wonderful service to humanity and this book will show you how to do it.

Michael Endacott
Deputy Director
Institute for Complementary Medicine
London, England

Acknowledgements

My sincere thanks go to the following for permission to quote from books, monographs, official publications and letters, and for information supplied:

Daphne Turner from her late husband Gordon's book, *A Time to Heal*; Ian Miller of the CW Daniel Company from the late Dr Ian Pearce's book, *The Gate of Healing*; Colin Page for his monograph on hypnotherapy; Michael Endacott; John Rolph; Ruth Rolph; Ken Fowler; Beryl Maskill; Kenneth Woodward; Jo Wallace, Secretary of the BAHA; Donald Copland, Administrator of the NFSH; Marcus McCausland; Tony Ortzen, Editor of *Psychic News*; Ray Branch of the Harry Edwards Healing Sanctuary; and Denis Haviland, CB, Chairman of the CHO.

In addition I must thank my wife, Karen, who acted as assistant proof reader in addition to all the other duties I heaped upon her.

1

Healing

*It was September and I was in my study at Castle Walk,
Doonfoot, Ayr, Scotland, looking out over the Firth of Clyde to
the mountains of Arran. I was worried.*

A gentle elderly lady, Grace Strathern, was coming to see
me as a patient, my very first. A chance encounter with
Grace had led her to ask, 'Will you give me healing?' Up
to that time I had not thought of being a healer. True, as a long-
time student of the paranormal, I had always had an interest in
healing as in other happenings that seemed to demand some
explanation. As a judo coach, I found I had a knack of being able
to put a vertebra back into place or perhaps rectify a shoulder
that was out … but a healer, me? You must be joking.

Grace had chronic arthritis of her hands. Her knuckles were
grossly swollen, as were her finger joints. The little finger of her
right hand was distorted and projected at an angle of about 60
degrees. Two doors down from our house lived Dr David
Johnson, a recently retired general practitioner. As I had never
acted as a healer, I thought it advisable to ask him along. With
Grace's permission, Dr Johnson examined her and gave his
opinion that there was chronic arthritis in both hands. His
prognosis was that no improvement could be expected.

Grace's knuckles were an enormous size; any attempt to
move the fingers brought her acute pain. She told me that she
had suffered from this condition for the past 25 years. One of
her main difficulties was the lifting of common household
objects; for example, she had to clasp a teacup between her

hands as she could not use the handle. Her fingers just could not bend.

Asking her to sit down, I moved behind her chair and tried to attune to her by placing my hands either side of her head, not touching her but keeping a short distance away. I asked her to relax and placed my hands on her shoulders. I looked out to Arran to try and induce the powerful peace of the mountains to flow into Grace. An instinctive act.

Now we came to the moment of truth.

I moved round to the front of Grace and asked her to extend her right hand while resting her elbow on the arm of the chair so as to minimise her discomfort. Placing my hands either side of her right hand, not touching her, I felt a tingling in my palms as if a power was passing from one hand to another and then being reflected back again, seemingly going through Grace's hands to my palms and bouncing back again. Odd. Grace remarked, 'My knuckles and joints of my fingers feel hot.'

Then the first and third fingers of her right hand straightened out ...

I am not ashamed to say that we both cried for joy.

Dr Johnson confirmed that there certainly was an obvious improvement but could not offer any medical explanation as to how it happened.

Such was my first experience as a healer.

So what was special about me? How had I been able to help Grace? Was I a religious person? No. Perhaps a very good, virtuous man who did not smoke or drink, and who had nothing but pure thoughts? Sorry again, I smoked, drank, ate meat (with great relish – usually horseradish), was certainly attracted to the opposite sex – in fact everything but an example of moral rectitude. As one of my long-suffering tutors once remarked, 'Butler, no one is completely useless, even the worst of us serves as a horrible example.' True.

That being so, what is healing? Your dictionary will give you a definition; I would say it is helping people to make themselves better. Dr Ian Pearce, then President of the World Federation of Healing, remarked to me when we were sharing the platform at a healing teach-in, 'All a doctor does is help a patient to get better, it is something inside the patient that completes the healing.'

So, what is healing? It is a natural function whereby we can help others who are not well to return to health. Some of us have 20/20 vision, others perfect pitch, all of us, unless we are blind or unable to use our hands, can draw and paint to some extent, albeit matchstick men or a coat of paint over the kitchen wall. So we can all heal. Of course our ability varies. Some can heal better than others, as can some draw better than others. Such ability as we have can be enhanced by training and experience. The use of proven techniques – those of which I am aware will be given in this book – will develop your potential so that you can maximise your ability.

How do you know if you have healing ability? Well, your first test is quite simple:

Hold your hands a little way apart in front of you.

Feel the flow of energy between your hands.

Have you got it?

If not, vary the distance a little and *seek* to feel the flow going from one hand to the other.

Now you should feel the flow. You do? Good.

Keeping your hands apart and maintaining the power flow, vary the distance between your hands so that the energy may feel like a piece of elastic. Stretch it until you feel the power flow diminish. This is the maximum. Now, slowly bring your hands together. At one point you will feel that maximum power flow again. Great, isn't it?

Not everyone, not even some quite successful healers, feels this power strongly in their hands, but most do. Some feel heat, others cold, a few just feel the energy flow. *You* will know when that power is there; that's all that matters.

At this point you require a partner. Notice I say 'partner', not 'patient' – I do not wish that you be unleashed on to the sick multitudes just at this point.

Ask your partner to sit down facing you and then to extend their hand. It is best that their elbow rests on the arm of a chair so that their hand, with fingers extended, can be relaxed.

Just say that you want to try an experiment.

Place your hands either side of their hand and move your hands outwards and inwards until you feel the power maximise as you did in the previous experiment. Got it? Good.

If you cannot sense any power, well, just lift your hands from either side of your partner's hand and energise as you did before. When you feel the power return, just place your hands either side of your partner's hand again. As you do so, be careful to keep the power going, but keep relaxed.

The power is there? Great. Maximise the power.

Ask your partner if they feel anything in their hand, any kind of sensation.

They may say, 'I feel hot/cold/pins and needles/a tingle'. They may, of course, say that they feel nothing at all. If they do, don't worry: about a third of my own patients feel nothing, yet many of them derive benefit from healing. Do not *suggest* that they should feel heat or a tingle; this defeats the experiment.

At this point you may feel you want to go just a stage further. The hand is not always the best way to test your healing power. With the further co-operation of your partner, ask them to sit back in the chair and relax. And this is what you do:

Stand behind your partner.

Place your hands, one at each side of their head, but not quite touching it.

Attune by letting the power flow through you.

If nothing seems to be happening, use the technique described above: lift your hands from your partner's head, get the power going and then place them on either side of the head. Adjust your hands until you maximise the energy.

Move your hands round your partner's head and see if the power varies. What I am saying is, if you are at the side of the head, say by the ears, try the forehead and the back of the head. Let your hands be like a radar set, seeking out the clearest, most powerful signal.

Ask your partner what reaction, if any, they feel.

If you have a partner who feels nothing at all, and yet you feel the power flowing through you, then obtain another partner and repeat the process.

I can hear you saying, 'It's all in the mind'.

You reckon? The technique of Kirlian photography demonstrates quite clearly and visibly the changes that take place in the structure of the human aura before and after healing. This was revealed to me by photographs taken at Leicester University. These showed clear changes in the force lines from my fingertips prior to healing and afterwards.

When I mentioned earlier that I was not an exceptionally good person, in fact far from it, you may have thought I was being unduly modest. I am not. I have known a lot of healers and they are a typical cross-section of the population: good, bad and, like me, somewhere in between.

Bad? Oh yes, by the standards of normal judgement. Take the case of Rasputin. This man was not as black as he is frequently painted, but there is no doubt that, in his youth at least, he was a lusty chap, not averse to living life very much to the full. The fact remains that he was a remarkable healer. The Tsarevitch, son of Nicholas II, the last of the Tsars, was a haemophiliac. Rasputin cured him on several occasions from dangerous haemorrhages. There are few healers who can stop bleeding instantly, but Rasputin certainly did. Yet I doubt if even Rasputin would have considered himself a 'good' man.

What is a good healer?

So what makes a good healer? The obvious criterion, I guess, is that a good healer is one who has an exceptional rate of success with the ills and ailments of patients. Such a person was most certainly Harry Edwards, the best-known healer in Britain. His name is a legend in healing circles and, even after his death, his work continues via his books. The Harry Edwards Sanctuary at Burrows Lea, Shere, near Guildford in Surrey, still carries on his work under the able direction of Ray and Joan Branch. Harry Edwards, who at one stage I was proud to have as my tutor, could fill the huge Royal Albert Hall in London with his healing sessions. Instant remissions could be seen by all. He was a most remarkable man, yet modest and always willing to help those in trouble. As is often the case with healers, he had seen more than his fair share of difficulties in his early days. After the First World War, when he had enlisted as a private but received a commission in the field and was promoted to captain, he had many business worries. By trade he was a printer but, on his own admission, was a poor businessman. At one time he held the London record for debt, having no less than 18 court warrants for debt outstanding at one time. Like many of us, he had a good education at the University of Hard Knocks.

At the age of 41, Harry discovered his gift of healing. He quickly established himself as a leading healer, and soon had more patients than he could see for contact healing. He then started practising absent (some call it 'distant') healing, where he attuned to patients regardless of where they lived or how far away they were from his home. In June 1944, a V1 bomb blew up his home in Balham, South London. He took a huge gamble and bought a large manor house called Burrows Lea in Surrey.

By 1948, Harry Edwards was receiving 3,000 letters each week from patients seeking his help. By 1974, the letters were over 10,000 in number each week and, in that year, the 15-millionth letter had arrived. Of course he had an army of helpers, the chief of whom were Ray and Joan Branch, and Olive and George Burton. And yet this man, who was doing so much, took time to tutor me, a novice healer, through the healers' course that he wrote with Gordon Turner, writing to me in his own hand. At the end of the course he was generous enough to award me a 100 per cent pass – I feel he may have been over-generous – and to invite me, along with other healers, to assist him at the Royal Albert Hall meeting. He was a great man of whom you will hear more shortly.

Let's go back a little. The question I asked was: what makes a good healer? Well, you have heard a brief outline of a great healer; but we cannot all be in the same class as Harry Edwards. I say again, everyone can heal. But there are people who are better healers than others. If I had to make a list of the common denominators among the most efficacious healers, my list would be:

Compassion
Empathy
Common sense
A wish to help

To these can be added other attributes such as humility, patience and kindness. Yet many healers do not have all of these virtues; I certainly haven't. However, I have listed four major, and three slightly lesser, character traits. Given that we all have healing ability, I suggest any two of the seven attributes will serve you in good stead as a healer.

I would like to explain what I mean with regard to the four major virtues; you may find that there is a variance from the dictionary definition.

Compassion is not *pity*. It is acceptance of people as they are, as one individual by another. It does not matter if the face is disfigured, that they are crippled or that they are suffering from cancer. We accept the person, warts and all, as *we* would like to be accepted in a similar situation.

Empathy is something we can give only if we have been through a similar experience. If people come to me and talk to me about their divorces, I can empathise with the pain and stress; I've been there. Or the loss of a parent, the stress caused by taking on too much, of having a heart attack – and then a second one. But I cannot empathise with a woman who has lost a baby. What a fool I would be if I said to such a person, 'I know how you must feel...'; 'Oh, and when did *you* last have a miscarriage?' would be a deserved reply.

Common sense seems a rather obvious blessing, but I include in this the ability to realise when we are not being told the whole truth by a patient. This does not mean that a patient may be deliberately telling you lies; just that matters are being put to you in such a way as to show the patient as an innocent party with little or no guilt for their condition.

A wish to help. This again may seem obvious, but there are some who feel it must be somewhat grand to be a healer (if only they knew). Others, thank heavens very few, are attracted by the power they think being a healer will give them over other people. Yet life is ever a joker; I have seen novices with these feelings change once they start healing. So motive is important.

What you have to do is to ask yourself, 'Why do I want to be a healer?' As a practical exercise, get a piece of paper and just write down why. Do it now or you will forget. Go on.

What were your answers? You see, if you are going to take such a step, you need a motive to keep you going when times get tough. If you are sure that you have been honest with yourself, then you have to decide what sort of healer you want to be.

Different sorts? Oh yes. Some regard a healer as a person giving all their free time to heal the sick. Not often, however. About 10 per cent of the healers that I know fall into this category, and only about 1 per cent heal full-time. The other 89 per cent vary from seeing ten patients a week to, perhaps, two a month. When we start healing, we may well find ourselves restricted to our own family and friends. If positive results are achieved, the word soon gets round; you will not have to advertise. However, I will save further comments until we come to the chapter 'Healing Others'. I just didn't want you to feel you had to have total dedication to the point where all your spare time is taken up with healing. It takes some of us like that, but not many.

Why do it? Let me give you the following example:

Dear Friends

To each and everyone who was at the meeting on 7th February when Pat Butler gave a talk on 'Spiritual Healing', please accept my sincere thanks for the kind thoughts given to me whilst he was easing the pain in my leg – which I assure you he certainly did. The relief was so great that for a long time after I seemed to be in a daze. It was so long since I had been free from pain that I could not believe it was true. Not only that but a great feeling of peace and contentment seemed to be all around – a wonderful experience I shall remember with gratitude to everyone concerned, all the days of my life.

On arriving home, this feeling of warmth and peace was still with me. For the first time since losing my beloved husband in 1970 I did not feel I was entering an empty home. Somehow it seemed that he, too, was sharing my happiness and a great wealth of love was surrounding us as it did whilst he was here with me on earth.

It was after 3 a.m. before I slept that night, not, as previously, because of pain, but because now the lack of it was so joyful. Whether it was because my thoughts were with my husband I don't know, but suddenly I smelled cigarette smoke and all the love in the world seemed to fill the room, so much, in fact, that tears of happiness just flowed until I fell asleep.

On waking at about 7 o'clock (more hours than I have slept continuously for longer than I can remember) this feeling was still with me and there was no pain in my leg – very unusual as the first thing I do is to reach for painkillers before getting from my bed.

I sincerely hope and pray that many more people can be helped as much and have the same experience as me. I do wish every success in the endeavour to find more healers in our group so that many more sufferers may benefit from this wonderful work.

(Signed) Gladys Dunkley

As a matter of interest, from this talk and demonstration a healing group was formed and several healers developed from the group, who, in turn, formed three more healing groups ...
Worthwhile?

Even if you only had one such healing a year, wouldn't it be worthwhile? Or even once in a lifetime?

I have files of such letters. A few are reproduced later in this book. These healings happened.

If my associates and I can do this, so can you.

I have been privileged to help many healers develop to their full potential. The methods and techniques that I have used are given here for your benefit and guidance.

They do work.

But so must you.

Test your progress 1

Back to practical matters. You remember how we tested to see how the energy flowed between our hands? Now we will put this to the test.

If one uses a partner who is anxious to help you, with the best will in the world they may report sensations that they may not really experience. For example, many people who have never had healing will have read reports of those who have and may say: 'Yes, I felt a gentle heat.'

So let us do an impartial, inanimate test.

Buy two flower bulbs. Try and get them the same weight (the Dutch, for example, grade their bulbs as if they used a micrometer) and plant the two bulbs in exactly the same-sized pots. Ensure that the same quantity of bulb fibre is used from the same container. You must have exactly the same conditions for both bulbs. On this test I recommend using hyacinths, as they have a reputation for growing in a consistent manner.

Place your planted and potted bulbs in such a way that both are in the same environment. Give them exactly the same amount of water and care.

The only difference in care you give the bulbs is that I want you, every night, to go up to the bulb that you select as the 'patient', and attune by placing your hands apart until you feel the energy flow.

Now place your hands over the chosen bulb and let the energy and love flow from you into the bulb. Envisage the bulb pushing upwards, forming a flower bud and flowering.

Carry on doing this and you will see an appreciable difference in the growth rate.

One word of warning. Do not curse or otherwise do down the 'non-patient' bulb. Just be objective in your treatment.

See what I mean? Your healing ability has been tested and actually proven.

If you have any doubts at all, ask someone else to examine the two bulbs and to say which is growing more strongly.

2

Develop Your Healing Potential

Now you are confident that an energy can be channelled through you, my task is to show you how you can use this power for healing others and yourself.

Each of us is a unique individual. The way we develop our healing ability is, therefore, a matter of personal choice. Some people prefer to join a healing circle or group as probationers. Such groups are under the guidance of experienced healers who accept, as part of their work, helping would-be healers. If you do not know of any activity of this nature in your area, then you can contact one of the organisations that are listed at the back of this book (see page 147). Go along and attend a session or two to see if this is the way you wish to progress and if you feel the particular group seems right for you.

There are many benefits to be gained from such an apprenticeship. You will be guided by experienced healers; patients will attend the meeting place for healing. You may be able to obtain probationary membership of the group which should, ultimately, allow you to obtain registration as a recognised healer of an organisation which is a member of the Confederation of Healing Organisations (CHO), the national body which represents the interests of British healers to various government bodies, including the National Health Service. In the USA, there is no equivalent to the CHO. In certain states, the right to heal the sick is jealously guarded, some might say restricted, by doctors, and legislation has been passed to limit the activities of healers. To counter this, some healers join a church, or indeed in some cases form a church, to carry out their ministrations under religious protection.

You could, however, pick up habits from other healers that may be fine for them but not for you. I well recall Harry Edwards telling me of a healer he was observing who, while giving healing to a patient, kept running his hands down his patient's body, bringing his hands together when he had completed his sweep. Then he would quite violently flick out his fingers away from the patient.

'What are you doing?' asked Harry.

'Oh, cleansing the aura of all this arthritis.'

'Well, be careful where you are throwing it. That last lump just missed my right ankle.'

Magnetic passes or any theatrical gestures are to be discouraged. In my opinion they do no good and, indeed, can unsettle the patient who starts to wonder what he has let himself in for. The healing process is a natural one and does need a relaxed attitude by both healer and patient.

By nature some of us prefer to be lone wolves rather than run with the pack. If you have a room at home that you can use to treat your patients, fine. Even if it is not possible to have patients visit you, owing, perhaps, to domestic arrangements, then you can always visit them. In the case of absent or distant healing, of course, no special room is needed.

Practical basics

The key to developing your healing potential to the full is your own attunement. While there are many systems of meditation and as many methods of attunement, let me describe an attunement for you which I have found to be of great benefit to myself and my students.

I would ask you to read, reread and then finally try out the attunement meditation on the following pages. While it may help you to close your eyes while attuning, obviously you cannot do this until you can remember the sequence. Further, the actual act of reading will, in itself, make your mind work at the very time when you are trying to relax. This can be overcome by either recording the attunement sequence on a tape recorder, making sure you leave plenty of time (I suggest the pauses below, but take longer periods between speech if you need them), or you can have someone read it to you slowly with the indicated pauses between each instruction.

Attunement – the key to healing

Sit down on a chair or the floor, whichever you prefer. Do not lie on a bed in case you fall asleep.

Close your eyes.
Breathe deeply, but in a relaxed manner. Release the stiffness from your body with every breath you exhale.

Pause for 10 seconds.

Let the tension drain from you. Let it drain from your head, neck, shoulders, down your arms and out through your fingers.

Pause for 20 seconds.

Now let the tension drain from your chest, heart, stomach, hips, down through your thighs to your knees, down the lower legs to your ankles and out through your feet and toes.

Pause for 20 seconds.

As you breathe, sense the beat of your heart; let it slow to a steady, slow throb. Sense the beat of your pulse at your neck and at your wrists. Imagine that the beat is in time with the pulse of the universe.

Pause for 20 seconds.

Let your whole self be in accord with the universal life force. Be at one with all. You are now at peace.

Pause for 15 seconds.

Bathe in this peace.

Pause for 15 seconds.

Gently, when you wish, let yourself return to the tempo of the day.

Now the tension you had before you started the meditation for attunement should have dissipated.

Pause for 10 seconds.

Wriggle your fingers, open and close them and let them rub on the palms of your hands.

Once you have practised attunement a few times, try sitting back and reflecting on the effect it has on you. It needs only a few minutes to go through the sequence, yet many people tell me it is like taking a spiritual bath.

I do not expect you to go through this attunement for every patient, but it will be of great assistance to you if you can undertake it before a healing session. As you become more experienced, you will find that you do not need as long before you become attuned. Eventually you may well be able to attune in a very short time indeed.

When you attune to a patient prior to healing, you need to be in a relaxed state. In this state you will be generating alpha rhythms from your brain instead of the beta rhythms that are generated by most people in a normal waking state.

Tests have proved that when an electroencephalogram machine is linked between a patient and a healer, then the alpha waves from the healer flood into the patient and the EEG pattern indicates an alpha state from the patient. In other words, the patient responds to and is affected by the state of mind of the healer.

You must, I am sure, have heard the expressions, 'Now we are talking the same language', or 'We're on the same wavelength'. That is just what you are doing when you attune to your patient.

Starting to heal

Now you are ready for the next step. Perhaps a quantum leap may be a better description. Why? Because you are about to try out your healing potential on a live patient. This is best done sooner rather than later – just as an experiment at this stage, nothing dramatic.

I would not recommend that you undertake the healing of a person with a serious condition, although this may be quite possible, but rather someone with a minor complaint.

For your first confirmation that your healing power can be used to help others, it can be helpful to work with a member of the family, a friend, or perhaps a colleague from work.

At this stage I am not suggesting that, even if the symptom of your patient is just a headache, you are going to cure what has caused the headache, but you are going to ease the tension and the pain.

The initial approach to your patient at this stage of your progress is important. Do not claim, 'I'm a healer' or, indeed, make any claim at all; far better to make a casual approach saying, 'I am sorry you have a headache. Will you let me soothe it away for you?'

Your manner should be one of gentle confidence.

If your patient agrees that you can try to help, then proceed as follows:

1 Ask your patient to sit on a chair: an upright one, not an armchair. Ask them to sit quietly for a minute or two while you compose yourself. Go behind them and place your hands lightly on your patient's shoulders. Ask your patient not to talk.

2 As you are standing behind your patient, carry out the attunement sequence that I described on pages 23–4. Since I hope you will have tried out the attunement many times prior to this, it should not take long to complete.

The act of attunement is, of course, the 'composing myself' that I described earlier.

3 When you feel attuned, raise your hands from your patient's shoulders and obtain the energy flow through them by holding your palms apart as you did in your first experiment (see page 13). *Up to this point do not concentrate on the headache of your patient.*

4 Now place your hands either side of your patient's head, a short distance away from the head. Vary the gap between your palms until you feel maximum power passing through their head from one hand to the other.

5 Visualise the energy flow dissipating your patient's headache just as water will swill away dirt. Do *not* try to will the headache away by your own *conscious* effort. It is not *you* who is doing the healing, it is the healing power flowing *through* you which is doing the job. At the end of the sequence I will explain why you must not use conscious effort, but for now you should just accept my word for it.

6 Move round your patient and vary the position of your hands, rather as if you are scanning in the way that a directional aerial works. Which is just what you are doing: you are seeking the strongest signal you can obtain. When you are on the maximum power feeling, or setting, if you prefer, ask your patient if they feel anything. They may say, 'A feeling of warmth', or 'cold', or 'tingling'. They may, of course, say they feel no reaction. If so, do not be concerned; many patients do not feel such a reaction, yet still benefit.

7 After a few minutes, ask your patient, 'How's your headache?' Whatever the reply, keep relaxed. If they say, 'Gone', then fine. If not, don't panic. Just place your hands on your patient's head and see if this makes a difference. You may no longer feel the energy flow yourself, but this need not matter. Except for spinal or joint injuries, I often do not touch my patients apart from the initial attunement that I obtain while placing my hands on their shoulders. However, Harry Edwards always used to put his hands on his patients. There is a strong suggestion of healing with the laying-on of hands, a ritual symbolism which can have a strong effect on both the healer and the patient.

8 When you feel that you have done all you can, let your hands fall to your sides and that will be an end to your first session. From the time you first placed the palms of your hands either side of your patient's head to withdrawing them, 10–15 minutes should have elapsed; 20 at the most. You will find that you may not be conscious of the passing of time while you are healing in quite the same way as when you are not.

I hope that your patient's headache has now gone or at least diminished. If it is still there, do not worry too much. My own failure rate is about one in three for reasons I will discuss in a later chapter.

Should you not have succeeded in your first attempt, try again with another patient; it could be someone with a stiff shoulder or neck. In such a case, use the sequence described above but, in addition, do place your hands on the painful area. We will go into the whys and wherefores in the chapter 'Healing Others'. Remember we are still at the stage of developing your healing potential.

Preserve your life force

The reason why you should not try to force any pain away from a patient has a simple explanation. By trying to *force* out a pain or disease you are *using your own life force.* This can be so debilitating for you that it could make you ill. I can illustrate this by describing what happened to me on my third healing attempt many years ago.

After my success with Grace Strathern and her arthritis, I was feeling more than a little pleased with myself. Note 'myself': hubris was certainly there. Not that unusual, as you may find, although I hope you will profit from my experience.

At work, one of my salesmen, called David, had a stiff shoulder and could hardly drive his car. I asked him into my office and said I would like to see if I could ease it for him. He agreed, expecting me to manipulate the shoulder. I did no such thing but stood behind him, attuned, and let my hands rest on his shoulders. After a short time, I moved both hands to the deltoid of his right shoulder. After a few minutes he told me that he felt a heat through his shoulder. When I removed my hands, David said, 'The pain's gone'.

Great. I was now ready to empty the hospital wards and heal the multitudes.

If only I had known.

I expect you are ahead of me. Pride certainly comes before a fall. For me it came about in this way.

There was a local shopkeeper, Brian, in Ayr in Scotland,

who had heard of the healing success of Grace Strathern. He had suffered for many years from a back complaint and asked for my help.

No problem.

After Grace and David, how could I fail?

I asked him to come to our house and, in my study, attuned. Nothing happened. I could feel no power between my hands, no energy flow. Right. I was determined that my patient should get better. So I carried on by concentrating on Brian's back, laying my right hand on the spot where he complained of the pain and my left hand on the front of his chest. I forced energy in. As I did so the strength drained out of my body.

I felt exhausted.

Brian exclaimed, 'Thanks a lot, I feel much better!' and left. I turned to my wife, Karen, and said, 'Gosh I feel weak', and staggered out to the back garden. Fortunately we lived across the road from the sea-front, so I was able to gulp in the good sea air. Yet, even then, I was unwell for several hours.

I contacted an experienced healer and he explained by telling me that what I had experienced was what he termed 'magnetic healing', whereby one person passes vital body energy to another. I do not commend it to you. In fact, the first thing I explain to my pupils is that they must let the healing flow *through* them. You must not generate your own life force and pass it to your patient because you feel so sorry for their condition. Compassion is one thing. Trying to force healing into a person by generating your own life force is quite another. The hardest thing would-be healers have to learn is that the power does not emanate from them. I know I have said it before, but I shall say it again, because it is the most important lesson that every healer has to learn. I learned the hard way. Profit from my foolishness, however well intended, and do not put yourself in this position.

Once I have attuned to the patient and envisaged their condition improving, I relax back into an objective state and let healing take its course. When I feel that the power is falling, then I gently disengage. The less concerned you are about the patient's condition, the more efficacious the healing will be.

That may sound strange, but think about it carefully and you will understand its truth.

If you are emotionally upset by the patient's condition, this is going to make you so uptight that your anxiety and resultant body tension may well impede the natural healing that is flowing through you.

Some of you may well be thinking, 'I hear what you say, but I'm not sure if I agree.' Well, let me give you an analogy. Suppose you are a surgeon. Every day you carry out operations. One day you are on duty when an emergency comes in and the doctor calls you down as he feels immediate surgery is required. You go down and find that the patient is your young daughter. How steady will your hand be when it is holding the scalpel? I maintain that unless you can be objective you will be unable to undertake a healing.

Now this life force, or vital body energy if you prefer, can leak from you as well as being deliberately pumped out. For example, have you ever visited someone in hospital who is very weak? This applies in particular to a patient who is getting on in years and whose powers of recuperation are not as great as they were. You sit there and chat and, after a while, the person you are visiting seems to perk up. Doubtless you feel quite pleased that your visit is doing them good. When you leave they may say, 'So pleased you came. I feel so much better.' All well and good. That is unless you are not all that full of energy yourself, for you may find that, quite unconsciously, the person you have been visiting in the hospital has been draining your life force. Well, if it is a relation or friend, you may feel it well worthwhile. However, if you are a hospital visitor or chaplain, you would soon be drained after visiting only a few patients. When you visit a patient in hospital as a healer, then these remarks do not apply as you will have attuned. But please refer to the advice in the Confederation of Healing Organisations' Code of Conduct (see pages 139–40) before practising healing in hospitals.

There is a most practical technique which I use to avoid letting my energy drain away. It has been known to generations of clergymen and others who have constant emotional demands made upon them.

As you sit down by the side of the bed of the patient, make a little steeple over your solar plexus (the navel *chakra* of the yogi) by letting the outside edges of your thumbs rest across your body at the bottom of the centre of your rib cage, while your little fingers lie tip to tip further down your stomach. Complete the steeple by raising your three other fingers so that they too are tip to tip, thus forming a steeple or pyramid. If you feel rather self-conscious, then a similar result can be obtained by just interlinking your fingers and placing your hands over your solar plexus.

There is perhaps only one set of conditions when this seepage of life energy can be of positive benefit to all concerned. This is when grandchildren are taken to visit their grandparents. Often the kids are so full of energy that they might well be deemed hyperactive. Old people tend to be rather low on energy and, quite naturally, soak up some of the surplus energy of the children.

Everyone is happy! The grandparents are recharged – just the way an undercharged battery benefits from a boost – and the parents get a rest while the kids are occupied with the senior citizens; they also benefit from the fact that some of the excess liveliness has been drained from their children. The children themselves are quite flattered that folk who have the respect of their parents take notice of them and like to have them around. This is one of the few situations in this life where everyone wins!

While we are on the subject of life force, there is something of which you must be made aware. There are certain folk in this world who are what I term leeches. Often they are unaware that they act in such a way, but there are also those who know quite well what they are doing. When in the normal course of the day you ask someone, 'How are you?', you do not expect a reply like, 'Oh well, bearing in mind the fact that I have had two heart attacks, have angina and dropsy plus hypertension, I struggle along'. This sort of person may well feed off you to become rejuvenated. As a healer you just do not need the drain that can come from this situation. When you are more experienced you can handle this sort of case; until then, steer clear.

Training and medical knowledge

There is a school of thought that maintains that healers are born, not made. It is a gift from God. No formal training or regulation is needed.

Maybe.

But I was not that good.

Once I knew I had healing potential, I rooted around and read every book on healing I could find. What a varied bunch they were. I had no idea until then that there were so many different approaches and viewpoints on the subject. With the exception of books by Harry Edwards and Gordon Turner, I could not find many that set out to help the would-be healer. However, help was at hand. I applied to join the National Federation of Spiritual Healers in England, who offered a four-part course which had been produced by Harry Edwards in collaboration with Gordon Turner. I worked away at the course and benefited from the sound advice given. The six papers set on anatomy and physiology, for example, ensured that a healer would not make elementary errors when talking to a patient, let alone when attempting to give healing.

As an example of what I mean, let me tell you what happened at a healing circle I was observing. A healer was told by her patient, 'I have acute discomfort in my right patella.' The healer immediately placed her hand over the patient's right scapula. If the healer did not know where the patella was, she could at least have had the wit to say, 'Just show me where you feel the pain'. It turned out that the patient was a medical student who assumed that the healer would know what he meant. I am quite sure he was not trying to catch her out as he was in genuine pain. Much embarrassment could have been saved by an elementary knowledge of human anatomy.

Many experienced healers say that any medical knowledge, however scant, can, in their view, hinder rather than help healing. The reason often put forward is that the job of the healer is to attune and pass healing on to their patients, nothing more. Indeed, some sincerely hold the view that a little knowledge can be a dangerous thing. I respect this view.

I am not suggesting that you should train to be a paramedic

but, as you gather, it is my opinion that you should at least know where the major organs and bones of the body are situated and, preferably, what functions they perform. In *A Time to Heal*, now sadly out of print (see page 154), Gordon Turner talks of his own early days and says, 'My slowly expanding knowledge of anatomy and physiology was a great help.'

So there you are. You must make your own decision. However, as standards demanded for membership of healing organisations are steadily rising, you may well find that formal qualifications may be expected in the future. We shall have to wait and see.

One thing is for sure. Healing cannot harm the patient. I tell my own students the following tale.

An old gentleman was very ill indeed. His wife noticed that his breathing had stopped. She telephoned the doctor who arrived within a few minutes. His examination confirmed that his patient was dead. The conversation went like this:

'I am very sorry, your husband has passed on.'

'I'll give him some chicken soup.'

'You don't understand. I fear your husband has passed on.'

'I'll give him some chicken soup.'

'Madam, he is dead. Chicken soup will not do him any good now.'

'It won't do him any harm ...'

Maybe healing is like chicken soup.

I hope by now you will have developed your healing ability to the point where you may have been able to help several people by easing their aches and pains. On a practical level you may find it difficult to get patients if you are not working in a group. Obviously you risk a snub if you just approach someone and offer healing: that is why I suggested family and friends may be your best first approaches. Mind you, should you find yourself short of patients to such an extent that you feel unable to progress, then after your regular attunement exercise, envisage someone who is ill coming to you for healing. If they are housebound or in hospital, imagine that, in your attuned state, you are visiting to give healing.

Should you hear any reports that the person you have been

thinking about has improved in health, do not claim to have had any part in this betterment. I suggest you maintain a low profile at this stage; it is satisfaction enough to know that you may have been able to help somebody.

Test your progress 2

I have stressed how vital it is for your proper attunement to take place before you attempt healing.

The more frequently you meditate for attunement, the less time it should take you to attune.

As a practical test, I want you to carry out a series of attunement meditations, one each evening, timing yourself with a stopwatch.

Start the watch as you sit down to attune. Do not *deliberately* set out to speed through the attunement, this defeats the object, but when you feel attuned, stop the watch.

Keep a record over a period of four weeks to see how the times compare. They should reduce, with the rate of reduction gradually levelling out, as it slows to a stop. Should the times not level out, then continue the test until they do so.

3

Benefit from Healing

When you are the patient of a healer there is a great deal that you can do to maximise the benefit you obtain from your healing sessions. Your basic attitude should be one of confident expectation. Your healer will try to attune to you and your condition, but you must help.

This chapter is addressed to the patient of the healer, but healers too will benefit from reading it and learning to look at the relationship from the other person's point of view.

Before your healing session

When you first meet your healer you will be asked to say why you need healing. It is essential that you be perfectly frank. My suggestion is that you give the following information:

1 What you feel is wrong with you.

2 If you have been to see a doctor, what diagnosis and prognosis has been made.

3 The treatment that your doctor or the specialist at the hospital has prescribed for you.

4 An outline of your own lifestyle and circumstances.

5 Any undue stress that you may have encountered prior to your illness, or family circumstances which may have upset the normal pace of your life.

6 Any material or emotional changes that you may have had of late. By this I mean a change or loss of job, money pressures, moving house, anything, in fact, that is a worry to you.

Do remember that everything you tell your healer as a patient will be kept in strict confidence and will not be passed on to a third party unless your permission has first been obtained.

In Britain, each healer registered with an association that is bound, as a member of the Confederation of Healing Organisations, to abide by a strict code of conduct designed for the protection of their patients. Extracts from the code are given elsewhere in this book (see pages 137–45).

It may well be, if you have not seen a doctor for your condition, that your healer feels you should take medical advice and may suggest you do so. If you are an adult, it is your right to refuse to do so if you wish. In this case your healer may well request that you sign a form confirming that you have been advised to seek help from a qualified medical practitioner.

Many healers like to talk to their patients in some depth before they start to heal. One reason for this preamble is that the healer is trying to establish a link between you both; another is to try and put you at your ease.

Should you have received healing before from another person, do please say so. On a personal note, I recall a certain lady at my clinic who, when she came to see me, started by saying:

'So pleased to meet you Mr Butler. I've heard so much about you and all the good work that you do.'

Suitably flattered, I smiled and indicated a chair. She continued.

'I've seen Harry Edwards, Gordon Turner and Ted Fricker, but they didn't do me any good.'

My smile faded. She had just named three of the most eminent and experienced healers in the country ... I am afraid that I did not succeed either. The lady was a hypochondriac whose hobby seemed to be visiting healers and, as I found out during the course of conversation, various homoeopaths, acupuncture practitioners and osteopaths. Her condition, on this occasion, was pain in the knees and ankles which, she felt, was due to arthritis. Since she was about 1.5 metres (5 feet) in height and, I estimated, weighed in at about 100 kilos (225 lb), I tentatively suggested that were she to lose some weight there might be less pressure on the joints bearing the load.

She turned puce and departed with the comment, 'You're the same as all the rest.'

Fortunately most patients do not have this demeanour.

The healing session

After a preliminary chat, your healer may ask you to sit on a stool rather than a chair. This is so they can move around you if they feel the need to change their position. There is no need to remove any clothing, except perhaps an overcoat, as clothes do not impede the healing force.

Your healer will then attune to you, hands being kept a little way from you. Many healers then lay their hands on the afflicted part of your body. Do not be surprised when, for example, if you have a pain down your leg, your healer concentrates on your back. It could well be, for example, that your sciatica may be caused by a prolapsed disc pressing on the nerve going down your spine. This may not be a conscious diagnosis, indeed a healer is not qualified to diagnose unless they are also a medical practitioner; the probability is that the therapist will run hands over the aura, the field extending a short distance from your body, obtaining a reaction which may indicate some strain or injury. In such a case, a referred pain may well be felt in your leg.

The time that your healer may spend with hands over or on you can vary from just a few minutes to 20. Do not worry about the period of contact. The amount of time spent rarely has any bearing on the efficacy of the treatment. Healing will continue until the healer feels that enough has been given, or that the healing energy passing through is waning.

I had a patient who came to see me complaining of migraine. I put my hands over her forehead and felt a quite exceptional burst of healing energy pass to her. After a short time I removed my hands and sat down behind my desk.

The patient looked at me and said:

'Is that all I get?'

'Sorry?'

'When I saw Mrs ..., she put her hands on for a good ten minutes.'

'How is your migraine?'

'Migraine? Oh, it's gone.'

After the healing

When your healing session has come to an end, your healer will ask how you feel now. Do give an honest answer. Do not say 'better' unless you mean it; you will only mislead your healer. Another appointment will probably be offered. If you accept, be sure to tell your healer if you find later you are unable to keep the arrangement.

On rare occasions there are instant remissions of an illness or condition. If you are fortunate enough to experience such a recovery, congratulations. But most patients improve steadily until the maximum improvement is obtained.

In my experience, benefit will be obtained within three visits. If not, it may well be that I am the wrong healer for the particular patient. In cases of this sort, perhaps one case in four, I will advise the patient to seek another healer and, if requested, I will suggest someone I feel may blend.

There can be after-effects to healing. The best one is that you feel much better, but there can be another side. It does sometimes happen that when you have had healing your condition may worsen within 48 hours or so. Do not become unduly alarmed about this if it happens to you. The reason can be that the healing has brought your condition to a head and, rather like a boil just before it is about to burst, the pain may be most acute prior to a marked improvement. Take any medication that you are using to alleviate any discomfort for what is normally a temporary state.

Keep in mind that healing is offered as a complement to orthodox medicine rather than an alternative. At least that is the policy adopted by most healers. Obviously you will have a deviation from this in a situation where the medical profession has said, in effect, 'Sorry, you will have to live with your condition.' The majority of patients I see tend to be folk who have tried orthodox medical treatment and found that their condition has not improved to the extent that they wish. A person with a cold does not go to a healer; if someone tried to make an appointment for such a condition I would not see them.

Now and again I encounter a patient who seems unable to benefit from healing. I do not know why this is so. My speculation is that it might be karmic (see page 111). The other thought that I have on the matter is that while a patient may seem to be overtly co-operating, perhaps subconsciously they may be rejecting healing. Fortunately these cases are rare; most patients I see benefit to varying degrees.

Payment

Now we come to the problem of money. Some healers, most in fact, will accept a donation if offered. Others who prefer not to do so have a charity box. One lady I know received enough donations over the years to pay for the purchase and training of many guide dogs for the blind. Should you wish to make a donation, ask if you can do so. All healers have expenses to pay, and in any case the offer is always appreciated. Any balance from expenses incurred by the healer will usually be donated to a charity.

There are a few professional healers who have no other means of livelihood except the fees they receive from patients. This can raise the hackles of the righteous who say that a person should not make money from what is a gift from God.

What, then, about a person with perfect pitch who becomes a piano tuner, or an artist with an ability to paint? Or a composer who, like Mozart, started composing at the age of five? We could continue with many examples. An athlete who has a natural ability, or for that matter, a person who has a vocation for the priesthood? Should all these folk not be paid?

If your healing is in such demand that you either have to reject patients or give up your job, what do you do? Professional healers I have known tend to be successful and highly experienced. Not many make a good living; most just get by. There is usually a fixed fee that you pay, but some professional healers may make a reduction for people in difficult financial circumstances. Should you decide to go to a professional healer, do ask what fee is payable, before making an appointment. A reasonable fee would be akin to that charged by an osteopath.

The human aura

You may have found it odd that your healer might have had his or her hands some distance from your body. The reason for this is that the healing, in this case, is being applied via your 'auric' field.

There is nothing mysterious about the aura. Every living thing has an energy field which can be measured and photographed. Prior to this century, such emanations were seen only by sensitives. Having said that, it is significant that medieval religious paintings frequently show a halo around the heads of saints, indicating the strong aura.

In 1908, Dr W J Kilner of St Thomas's Hospital in London discovered that, by treating glass screens with chemicals, a haze could be seen round the human body. This work continued until Kilner published his initial findings in 1912. There was a mixed reception. However, he carried on with his experiments, publishing further findings in 1921. His results were confirmed by Oscar Bagnell, a Cambridge biologist, and author of *The Origins and Properties of the Human Aura.*

It was not until after the Second World War that we, in the West, became aware of progress that had been made in the USSR by two Russian researchers, Valentina and Semyon Kirlian, who found that energy fields around the human body (the aura) could be photographed. This process is called 'Kirlian photography' in popular approaches to the subject, but the term 'radiation field photography' is used by many researchers.

Modern research has mushroomed, with scientists all over the world working on energy fields, L-fields, T-fields and biofeedback techniques. As early as 1949, the Kirlians with their high-frequency photography were able to illustrate that the leaf of a diseased plant had a weak aura whereas that of a healthy leaf had a strong one. 'So what?', you may ask. The 'what' is that there was no visible sign of disease on the leaf with the weak aura. The illness of the plant had been diagnosed ahead of time. Details of the work undertaken by the Kirlians are given in *Psychic Discoveries Behind the Iron Curtain* by Sheila Ostrander and Lynn Schroeder. This work and its implications make up a most specialised subject in itself with which the rest of this book could be filled.

'So what's new?': that was the cry of the clairvoyants, or many of them at least, when the scientific world demonstrated its new toys. Clairvoyants had been seeing auras and disease in and around people for centuries. Some even have the ability to see diseased organs.

During the 1960s, it was my good fortune to know Ena Twigg, the eminent healer and medium. She told me she not only saw the aura of a person in full colour, but had been able to do so from childhood. In fact it came as quite a shock to her when she found that other people did not have the same ability. Ena would say to me, 'Oh dear, your aura's dull today; you're feeling depleted, are you not?' She was right. Once she said, 'Gosh, that's an angry red in your aura – what happened?' What had happened was that a taxi nearly knocked me down on a pedestrian crossing on my way from the underground station to the College of Psychic Studies.

While Ena Twigg may be as good as, or better than, any machine so far available, it is not practical to have someone of her ability on standby in every hospital, clinic or surgery in the country. Because of this, if for no other reason, the experienced healer should try to co-operate with these developments rather than adopt a Luddite attitude. Most of us older healers are, perhaps, even with the best will in the world, a little apprehensive of technical and electronic innovations.

A final word on the aura. I had my second heart attack on 23 November 1985. Ten days before the attack my aura was tested by one of my students at a class on the paranormal. My auric field was shown as extending 53 centimetres (21 inches) from my body, as indicated by the machine the student used.

When I returned to the class my aura was measured again. This time it was just 10 centimetres (4 inches).

The fact that I am still here five years later is due in no small way to the combination of skilled medical care I obtained from my doctor and the loving healing so generously given by my wife and my many healer friends. I firmly maintain that medical attention and healing can work well together.

Illness and state of mind

I have no doubt that much disease is caused by our own actions and attitudes of mind. The term used to describe this type of illness is a psychosomatic disease. At one time, not so many years ago, the word psychosomatic was unacceptable to many members of the medical profession. Even now some medics treat the concept of psychosomatic illness merely as a mental state of the patient that may have an effect *on* a disease rather than as a prime *cause* of illness. Attitudes are changing though. For example, stress is recognised as a major contributory factor in certain diseases. Be that as it may, doctors, in the main, translate 'psycho' as 'mind', or the subconscious or unconscious mind. Many healers use the word 'psycho' in another context. The word is derived from the Greek *psukhe*, meaning spirit or soul. So when a healer uses the word psychosomatic it may well be in the context of soul sickness.

I am grateful to Marcus McCausland, founder of *Health for the New Age*, for permission to quote from his paper of February 1975. The views Marcus expresses are in accord with my own, and I know from my healing work that the extract which follows is true:

> To become a complete and whole person, a patient requires to achieve an understanding of himself and a maturity and wisdom which he may not previously have possessed. He will then be able to reassess his values and the material values in his day-to-day existence. This will then cause a change in his way of life and in his attitudes, and all his levels will then begin to slot into place in an harmonious whole. For a healer to be able to help with these changes, there has to be contact from the inner self of the healer to the inner self of the patient.

This happens on a completely different unconscious level to that between the subconscious of the two individuals. When the healer displays the highest form of love (completely selfless love) with compassion and sympathy, the patient reacts in a very special way and may begin to realise that the pain and suffering which led up to this moment in his life were the means, or key, which opened the door to a beautiful new world which was awaiting – the door which permits the soul, which was imprisoned within himself, to emerge and start growing. When the change starts, true healing of the whole person can begin. There may be occasions where the self-to-self contact is made immediately, and a miraculous (so-called) healing occurs. This is not the norm by any means.

In general, healing takes place over a long period and involves a lot of heart-searching and effort on the part of the patient. Without this higher level of healing, it is likely that the patient may revert to his previous state, whatever it may have been, of pain and suffering, although the manifested symptoms may be different.

What Marcus McCausland says applies to the healing in depth that changes a person's life completely. It is rare, but it happens, and when it does, all the effort and sacrifices made are worthwhile.

The damage that stress can do was well illustrated by Gordon Turner in *A Time to Heal*.

Gordon was ill but, rather than go to hospital, felt it his duty to attend the summer school of the National Federation of Spiritual Healers in the UK of which he was chairman. Two days after the ending of the summer school while he was healing a patient he reports the following:

At twenty-five minutes past five on the afternoon of Wednesday the 28th September 1966, I felt a sudden loss of mobility in my left hand. Ironically, I was attempting to heal an elderly man suffering from the after-effects of a stroke. I asked him to excuse me and left the room. My left leg dragged and my speech was slurred.

I had been aware for several months that my blood pressure was too high. I should have gone to hospital for tests, but there was so much to do ...

> At twenty-five minutes past five I was totally indispensable.
> At twenty-six minutes past five I was effectively dispensed with.
> Just like that. All it took was one little cerebral thrombus.
> One little blood vessel, which could not stand up to the
> unreasonable pressures to which it had for so long been
> subjected, brought my life's work crashing down about my feet
> like so much powdered plaster.

One of Gordon Turner's favourite sayings after his stroke was, 'Life is leasehold'. An important point. Most of us go through life as if it were freehold. And yet, when you think about it, life certainly *is* leasehold; the only trouble is that, unlike most leases, you are not told at what date the lease is up.

We all need some stress in our lives to make us function: you do, I do. The point is that you may be able to take a much higher level of stress than I can. Again, if you are the type of person who expresses feelings by shouting, swearing or crying, you are less likely to suffer from stress than the person who suffers in silence. The introvert swallows anger, sorrow and hurt. Not that it goes away. The process is rather like receiving a demand for payment from your local income tax office. You can take action by paying the demand or disputing it, or you can pop it away in a drawer in the fond hope that it will go away, or perhaps you think if you cannot see the demand it can no longer worry you. Not so. Sooner or later the red demand comes, then the bailiff comes to call.

In the same way, you can pop away, or file, your angers, sorrows and frustrations in your unconscious. But they will lie there. And they will fester away until they can no longer be contained. Then they will explode and you may well have a stroke, heart attack, hypertension or kindred discomforts.

Certainly the late Dr Ian Pearce, Vice President of the Suffolk Healers Association in England, told me several times of his firm conviction that stress was a major factor in cancer. I will be coming back to Dr Pearce's views later in the book but in the meantime I would mention a personal experience bearing out Dr Pearce's views.

I became convinced that emotional disturbance was a major contributory cause of cancer in many cases when both my father and uncle died from cancer within a year or so of having marital difficulties. Among my patients at least half who had cancer were subjected to extreme emotional pressure. In some cases it was as though the person had lost the will to live and pushed the self-destruct button.

I have permission from one of my patients to publish her experience of healing after she had cancer and the specialist wanted to remove a breast. Prior to the operation she came to see me and, after a rather hectic four-hour session which involved her husband as well, we thought we had pinpointed the emotion that caused her cancer. Her letter reads:

Dear Pat,

Four months ago I came to you, very worried about my state of mind and concerned about a small lump in my breast which subsequently proved to be cancer. I was, I believe, about as low as it is possible to get but after each meeting with you I became a little better until at last I began to shake off the awful depression which had made me so ill and which in my opinion was the cause of the cancer.

I can never thank you enough for saving my life, and if that sounds dramatic it's nevertheless true, because I am now happy and content. I have been given a second chance and this time I will not fail because I've learned and am learning all the time that I have a purpose in life and a whole new meaning.

Condensed into these very few words it all sounds very simple, but I know that I was a great trial to you at first and I really appreciate everything you've done for me and those concerned with me.

Thanks to you I am a complete person again (boobs and all). Thank God I came to see you when I did. If I can ever help anyone in doubt, as I was, I will be only too willing to talk to them and give them my assurance that healing can help them – it certainly has in my case. Bless you Pat and keep up the good work.

Love from

Beryl Maskell

To illustrate my point, let us take another case with a follow-up ten years on:

Dear Pat,

I write to thank you most sincerely for the healing treatment which you have given me over the past five months.

I came to you on a recommendation at a time when I was feeling far from well following a month of almost daily radiotherapy treatment, subsequent to an operation at the end of May for the removal of a cancerous growth from the left side of my neck. It was two days after your first healing treatment that I noticed an improvement, but didn't immediately relate this improved feeling to the treatment I had received from you. From that time on, however, I improved tremendously and I now feel fit again, doing a full day's work and enjoying life to the full.

My present hospital visits as an out-patient are at present bimonthly and if I continue to progress satisfactorily, as I expect to, the periods between visits will gradually be extended. I have not had any further medical treatment since I finished the course of radiation; my only treatment has been your healing treatment, which I value highly and can never thank you enough for. I shall always feel deeply grateful to you, not only for the treatment itself, but also for giving me faith and hope for the future.

Once again, my grateful thanks for everything Pat, and long may you continue in your wonderful service to others.

Yours very sincerely

Ken Fowler

Every year Ken and I exchanged Christmas cards and he would sometimes send me a postcard from a holiday visit or drop me a few lines. On 6 December 1988 I received the following letter:

My dear Pat,

I am pleased to report that I am very well, in fact so well that on the 5th February last the hospital doctor decided he didn't want to see me any more. Wasn't that good news? As you can guess I was over the moon.

I never lose sight of the fact that I received so much help from you in those early days, Pat, for which I shall be eternally grateful. I know much of my success is down to you.

Bye for now, Pat

Ken Fowler

I have not included these letters to show what a good or clever person I am. They are published so that you too can benefit from healing. In both cases the patients were prepared to work along *with* me. They were able to root out what may have caused the disease by a change in attitude but mainly by seeking a second chance. How?

A Second Chance

To benefit from healing in depth you must be prepared to make a fresh start. This involves asking for forgiveness from those whom you have hurt, be it by intent or when you do something without thinking which did not work out too well. You also have to forgive those who have hurt you.

If you, as an individual, try to impede the flow of life, you will be pushed aside, getting bruised and hurt in the process. If you decide to flow along with the river you can succeed.

The first thing to do is get a large piece of paper. Think back as far as you can to your earliest childhood. Trace your progress through life by writing down:

> Any hurt that anyone has done to you.
> Any action that has caused you to suffer.
> Each time you felt unfairly or unjustly treated.
> Any situation that caused you to resent either the person concerned or the circumstances involved.

Having done this, and please do not hurry the process, go slowly through each item and fully forgive each and every one.

Next, take another piece of paper and write down:

> Any action in your life of which you are ashamed.
> Anything that you have said or done which has hurt someone, even though you did not intend this.

Mentally ask the forgiveness of each person, alive or dead. To be effective this system *must* be carried out in depth and your forgiveness must be genuine. Once cleared, do not go back and think 'if only' or 'I wish I had'. Let it go. You have now learned the lesson. Having done this, *burn the papers*. Do not reread or show to, or discuss them with *anyone*.

You now have a new start.

You have wiped clean the floppy disc containing the nasty parts of your memory. In the process you will find some of the unconscious contents come back into your conscious memory and can also be released.

You may find that as you work through the sequence I have called 'A Second Chance' there will be people whom you are unable to forgive. If so, do not agonise for too long but move on to the people or events that you can forgive. This will reduce the overall internal pressure. Mind you, you will have to return to your sticking point(s) later. I suggest that, once you have gone through 'A Second Chance', you do the sequence again a week or ten days later. If you are still unable to forgive any person or situation (i.e. 'an act of God'), work through it at monthly intervals until you feel you are completely free of the dross.

You may find, eventually, that there is still one major injustice that has hurt you so much that you just cannot forgive. What you are experiencing as an injustice may be karmic: I deal with this aspect in Chapter 8 (see pages 110–11).

Even after you have cleared out all the dross and climbed the mountain of forgiveness, you will, in the course of everyday living, collect further resentment. I know I do. So my advice to you is to work through 'A Second Chance' at least once a year and release that resentment and unseen stress that can build up and indeed, unless you are a saint, will build up.

When I first wrote 'A Second Chance' many years ago, I sent copies to several magazines and it was published in five. I waived copyright as I wanted as many people as possible to benefit from the exercise as my own patients have done.

Reprints have reached me from several sources all over the world. It is a practical method of self-help which should be available to all.

You may feel that I am putting too much emphasis on psychosomatic illness and stress. I do not think so.

In *The Gate of Healing* (see page 154), Dr Ian Pearce writes:

In my thirty-five years' experience as a practising doctor I have
been gradually brought to the view that a very large proportion
of the diseases from which we suffer are not random
occurrences, inflicted on us from without, but are created by
ourselves through wrong patterns of emotion and faulty
attitudes of mind. In my experience some three-quarters of the
physical diseases brought to me in my consulting room were
'psychosomatic' in origin.

Dr Pearce gives six examples in his book of such cases. I
have selected just one to illustrate the point he makes:

Bob was a man in his early fifties whom I had known for some
twenty-five years. He was a cheerful extrovert, of whom I had
seen remarkably little apart from an occasional bout of
influenza. One night in early spring he appeared in the
consulting room and sat down in front of me with an
extremely long face. Something was obviously very wrong.
    'Doctor,' he said, 'I think I am getting rheumatism.' He
held out his hands for me to see. Sure enough there were the
early signs of rheumatoid arthritis. The swollen knuckles and
wrists and distorted joints all told a familiar story to the
experienced eye. What was surprising was that Bob was not the
sort of person who one would have expected to develop this
disease. After a time one learns to recognise that certain types
of personality are particularly prone to develop certain types of
disease and Bob was not the rheumatoid type. Recognising that
rheumatoid disease tends to be associated with the resentful,
worrying, obsessional type of personality, to whom the
problems and difficulties of life always seem too hard to
overcome, I started to talk to Bob about the relationship
between the mind and disease. He pulled me up short. 'But I
don't worry doctor. You know I'm not a worrier.' This was
certainly true. Bob was not the worrying type. 'Sure,' I replied.
'I know you don't worry, Bob. But there are an awful lot of
emotions besides worry which can interfere with your body.'
    I spoke of the various negative emotions; envy, hatred,
resentment, jealousy, discontent, and what might be loosely
lumped together in the classic phrase as 'all uncharitableness'.

Bob sat very quiet for a space, obviously turning something over in his mind.

'Well now doctor,' he replied, 'I'll tell you something. You know I used to work for …' and he mentioned the name of a local public utility company for whom he worked.

'Yes.'

'You know that last January we were all amalgamated?'

'Yes.'

'Well, one day I was walking through the office and I happened to see on the table my personal file. Now I know I shouldn't have done this, but I just couldn't resist having a look inside to see what they said of me. And there, in capital letters across the top, and in red ink too, I saw the words "No potential for promotion here" and I have been so angry that they should do this to me, and after all these years, that I haven't been able to get it out of my mind.'

'And when did this happen?'

'About three months ago.'

'And when did your rheumatism start?'

'About a month later.'

'Well there you are,' I said. 'You've been so eaten up with resentment over this slight that it has been burning up your body. That is what caused your trouble.' I then proceeded to apply some correction. 'Now tell me, are you any worse off as a result of this?'

'No. I'm doing exactly the same job, and I'm getting the same money.'

'Would you have expected to have been promoted, if there had been no amalgamation?'

'Oh no, there would have been no room in the establishment.'

'And you were not thinking of going out and looking for a job which would have paid you more money?'

'No. I was quite content, and there was enough for my requirements.'

'So – you are no worse off. You're doing the same job, and you're getting the same money, and you are not thinking of going out and looking for a rise. And,' I added, 'you know there is always the possibility that if you had been promoted you might have found the extra load of responsibility too heavy to carry.'

'Oh,' said Bob. 'I never thought of it like that.'

So he left the consulting room with a prescription for

some butazolidine and some aspirin and a lot to think about. When he returned a month later for a follow-up, I was away on holiday and he saw my partner.

It was not until six months later that I again saw him, and it was not in the consulting room. I had gone out for a haircut and there, swapping jokes with the barber, I found Bob looking a picture of health and in the best of spirits.

'Hullo, Bob,' I said. 'How are you?'

'Me? Oh, I'm fine, doctor.'

'What? No rheumatism?'

'No, doctor. Look.' He stretched out his hands towards me. 'It has all gone away.'

It had. Bob's hands were completely normal, and there was no trace of the disfiguring arthritic deformities. In the language of my profession, Bob's condition had undergone a spontaneous regression. That generally means that a healing has taken place and the doctor has not the least idea of how to account for it.

What, in fact, had happened was this. Bob had switched off the injurious flow of energy resulting from his feelings of hurt pride and resentment, and the natural healing power of his body, aided a little by the anti-inflammatory powers of aspirin and the butazolidine, which he had been given, had done the rest. Bob was fortunate. He had changed his patterns of thought before the physical damage was irreversible.

I think you will agree that Dr Pearce has described a classic case of illness with psychosomatic origin.

From this you will see what an opportunity you have with 'A Second Chance' to counter psychosomatic disease by dealing with the stress factors that, either in themselves or in part, contribute to illness.

A basic concept that you have to accept to benefit from healing fully is that you are the one responsible for your own health. Health services provide many benefits to people who otherwise could be without adequate care and specialist advice. But there is another side.

You may think your doctor is responsible for your health. Not so. You are. Your doctor, certainly, is the one you visit if you are not well, and I have no doubt that he or she will do everything possible, within the resources and time that can be allocated to you, to deal with the symptoms that you show. But, and here's the rub, if you carry on in this way of life that may have caused or at least contributed to your illness, you cannot blame your doctor if you do not get better.

Let me take an extreme and rather obvious example. If I am fool enough to drink two bottles of whisky a day and develop cirrhosis of the liver, I only have myself to blame. Yet, perhaps, just a tot in the evening may be of real benefit.

Health is a positive state of mind and body. What you eat and drink, your lifestyle, how you deal with stress and, I venture to say, your philosophy of life, have a profound effect upon your health; far more than most people will acknowledge.

Self-healing techniques

We can return now to the practical self-healing techniques that you can undertake in addition to any healing or medical treatment.

Self-healing meditation
Your meditation for attunement was given on pages 23–4. Now I want you to move on to the self-healing meditation.

Sit down in a comfortable position on the floor or in a chair, whichever suits you best.

Control your breathing until a deep, regular, soothing rhythm is obtained. Breathe in this manner during the whole meditation.

In your mind, build a seashore. You are on a beach of golden sand, looking out over a calm blueness. Keep this image.

Pause for 20 seconds.

The cloudless sky is a lighter shade of blue than the sea.

The sun shines down, the slanting rays mixing with the sea to give a reflection of varied hues of gold and blue.

Pause for 20 seconds.

Such is the combination of colours that you now have from sun, sea and sky, that you know a healing power is ready, waiting for you to absorb all that you need.

Pause for 20 seconds.

Move into the glorious, golden, blue light that is now ready for you. Soak up the healing power of the universal life force which now pervades your whole being. Bathe in the beauty and healing tide which engulfs you.

Pause for 60 seconds.

Gently, slowly, move backwards out from the glorious light as it gradually fades.

Pause for 20 seconds.

You are now back on the shore, relaxed and rejuvenated by the healing power retained in your body.

Pause for 30 seconds.

Gradually come back to your waking state. Blink your eyes and gently wriggle your toes and fingers.

This meditation will give you a positive benefit but do not undertake it more than once a day.

There are many systems of meditation which employ various techniques. The best that I have encountered for either healers or patients are those of Gordon Turner, whose meditations I use. In Britain, many are available on cassette; check your local bookshop for others.

In addition to meditation and 'A Second Chance', we have yet a further method of self-healing to try. This is visualisation.

Let us take one of the worst situations that you can encounter. Suppose you have cancer of the breast. There is a lump and it has been diagnosed as malignant. In addition to the other methods given in this chapter, I suggest you use the visualisations I give below before you resort to surgery. Combine these with a visit to a healer, or, should this not be possible, obtain absent healing.

White knight visualisation

Envisage the cancer cells as black knights. Summon up all the resources of your body to crush and defeat them. Visualise the healthy cells of your body who are about to do battle as white knights who cannot be defeated.

In the battle the black knights are broken, killed and crushed. Their remains are passed from your body with other waste matter. Nothing is left of them.

After each visualisation, carry out the self-healing meditation given earlier (see pages 52–3).

Laser visualisation

Whatever the seat of your disease, whatever decay is taking place, *burn it out.*

You have at your command a laser gun of greater power than any machine built in this world.

Focus on the area of the disease.

Fire your laser. The scorching power burns out and consumes the malignant cells while strengthening the normal cells in your body that are helping you.

Combine this exercise with the healing meditation.

Wholeness visualisation

An organ of your body is under attack.

Bathe the area in the light and power you obtain from the healing meditation.

Let the cells which have been invaded be converted to healthy tissue by the light and power of the universal life force in which you have been bathing and which is now filling every part of your body.

Such is your total absorption that your higher self releases your own inner healing power in full force.

You feel the upsurge of new life, a rejuvenation.

The type of visualisation that you choose will depend on the kind of person you are. Once you have understood the concept, then you will be able to devise your own individual visualisations.

You now have three powerful self-help techniques to use: 'A Second Chance', meditation and visualisation. Healing and medical treatment can be partners with all three methods.

Test your progress 3

This chapter has been about obtaining benefit from healing. When you have improved and your health is restored, show your gratitude by helping someone else. You do not have to be an active healer to use this technique.

Please read through with care the meditation I am now going to give you. It may seem like the self-healing meditation, but there is an important addition.

In your mind, build a seashore. You are on a beach of golden sand, looking out over a calm, blue sea. Keep this image.

Pause for 20 seconds.

The cloudless sky is a lighter shade of blue than the sea. The sun shines down, the slanting rays mixing with the sea to give a reflection of varied hues of gold and blue.

Pause for 20 seconds.

Such is the combination of colours that you now have from sun, sea and sky, that you know a healing power is ready, waiting to be absorbed.

Pause for 20 seconds.

Now you are ready to move into the healing light, but this time think of a person who is unwell and in need of healing. Imagine that person by your side and, taking your companion by the hand, move into the universal life force which awaits. Once there, after ensuring that your friend is absorbing the healing, slowly withdraw to the shore so that your companion benefits from all the power that is available.

Pause for 60 seconds.

As the healing light slowly fades, ask your companion to rejoin you on the shore.

Pause for 20 seconds.

Return to your normal state. Blink your eyes and gently wriggle your toes and fingers.

4

Healing Others

*What are we, as healers, trying to do? The normal reaction of
most healers will be, 'Why, to heal others of course, and to
make them better'. Yes. I quite agree, but what are we trying to
heal? The symptoms? The pain? The discomfort? All this, yes.
But what should be our ultimate aim?*

I suggest to you that what we are trying to do is to heal the
whole person: the 'holistic approach' as it is often called.
The holistic concept, as I understand it, is that one treats the
person rather than the disease. In the last chapter I quoted Dr
Ian Pearce from his book, *The Gate of Healing*. Let me now,
looking at the situation from the viewpoint of you as a healer
rather than a patient, pursue the matter. The holistic attitude is
vital to our function as healers.

Dr Larry Dossey wrote a book entitled *Beyond Illness* (see
page 154) which I was asked to review for the NFSH publication,
Healing Review. This I did and the review was subsequently
published. I quote extracts from my own review of Dr Dossey's
book as follows:

> I am sure that every healer can benefit from reading this book
> by Dr Dossey whose depth of perception on the need for
> fundamental rethinking on the basic concepts of health and
> illness may be considered iconoclastic by his fellow physicians.
>
> Larry Dossey, former Chief of Staff, Dallas City Hospital, is
> now engaged with the Dallas Diagnostic Association.
>
> In his book he has combined his practical experience
> with an insight rarely seen in medics. He quotes a figure of

10 per cent as the percentage where medical intervention is dramatically successful, and 9 per cent where some success is obtained. He asks, 'But what of the 80 per cent of persons for whom modern medicine is not very helpful? It is largely from the needs of this group that the holistic health movement has evolved. Its emphasis, unlike the orthodox approach, is on the psyche, not the soma, and, according to some advocates, on the spiritual as well. Wholes, not parts, are said to be the most important. There is great importance attached to the health-creating effects of lifestyle, exercise, nutrition, and the self-regulatory techniques designed to annul the noxious effects of stress on the body.'

Another quote: 'Every physician knows that there is a limit to therapies of every sort, beyond which they become downright meddlesome, interfering, even dangerous, the progenitors of one of the commonest diseases of our day, that of iatrogenic illness (illness caused by the doctor). It is the amazing intelligence and strength that is part of the body, and that is part of the world encompassing the body, that makes heroes of surgeons and seers of diagnosticians.'

With regard to holistic medicine, Dr Dossey does not argue with the concept, but points out that a typical response from a hard-working doctor may well be, 'Where in the name of everything holy does it say that a physician is to be more than a healer of sickness?' He goes on to say, 'Take for example the case of several deaths occurring in an holistic clinic which promoted enema therapy (colon cleansing), a popular health-care technique. Owing to failure to properly disinfect the enema equipment, a deadly micro-organism was spread from patient to patient ... Of the persons infected six died – all from a technique, opponents would say, there was no justification for in the first place – and adding, in derision, that it is no better to die holistically than any other way.'

Even-handed Dr Dossey provides the viewpoint of a registered nurse who gives a personal account: 'I did not pass Go. I went directly to jail – the hospital bed. Each physical examination left me in worse shape – all that pressing and poking was not helping my pain or my mind very much ... it was also evident that the attending physician wasn't too sure what was going on either.'

Later in the book a Harvard doctor is quoted as saying: 'An important principle is the laying-on of hands – a practice that is rapidly atrophying because physicians are too busy with the laying on of tools.'

When talking about spiritual healing, Dr Dossey begins with St Augustine's reminder, 'Miracles do not happen in contradiction to nature, but in contradiction to what we know about nature'. He continues: 'My own inclination as a physician is to acknowledge it as a special form of healing, for I cannot dismiss as deranged all the persons who have written about this phenomenon and who have claimed to have experienced it themselves.'

Some of you may have cause to wonder at certain of the fringe activities that are promoted as 'alternative therapies'. I must say that certainly I have myself. In this regard Larry Dossey makes a point that should be carefully considered prior to the reflex action of rejection we may now be conditioned to make. He writes: 'The holists, on the other hand, may object that the insertion of levels may sunder man's oneness and unity. I suggest that what is more likely to be sundered by a rational map of the territory of reality is not one man's oneness and unity with the cosmos but the undisciplined, sloppy metaphysics that have defiled the perfectly legitimate philosophy of holism and which have greatly distorted the disciplined thinking that has always lain at the heart of great mystical paths.'

So there you have it. Perhaps, as healers, some of us tend to throw out the baby with the bath water, the more brain-washed of us chanting, like the workers in George Orwell's *Animal Farm*, 'Holistic and alternatives good, medicine bad'.

The soul in the healing process

It is a commonly held view that the concept of psychosomatic illness is one that has recently come to light. No so, for in 380 BC Plato wrote in the *Republic*:

> The cure of a part should not be attempted without treatment of the whole. No attempt should be made to cure the body without the soul, and therefore, if the mind and body are to be healthy, you must begin by curing the mind. This is the first thing. Let no one persuade you to cure the head until he has first given you his soul to be cured. For this is the great error of our day in the treatment of the human body, that physicians first separate the soul from the body.

59

More than one author has used this quotation. Mind you, if you popped along to your local doctor and asked him or her to cure your soul, I fear you would get short shrift. Your doctor might urgently telephone the local psychiatrist who, in turn, would doubtless tell your doctor that the soul was not under his or her jurisdiction but lay, more correctly, under that of the local minister.

Given that in this day and age more doctors accept the concept of psychosomatic illness, there is the problem of the relationship, if any, between you as a healer and the medical profession.

Try to be objective. Take a look at the situation from the viewpoint that you might take as a doctor. After an extensive education you apply to become a medical student. There are far more applicants than places, so you have to be outstanding to be accepted.

During your intensive and demanding studies, should you fail any examinations you are 'put back' and have to resit the examination. Some medical students cannot take the pressure or meet the standards, or find that they do not have a vocation for medicine. So they drop out.

If, after years of training, you do manage to qualify as a doctor, you have still to undergo practical experience in a hospital before you can contemplate becoming a general practitioner.

Should you wish to become a specialist, then several more years of study lie ahead of you.

So, here you are, a doctor who has spent many years of intensive study and apprenticeship, confronted by a case where a healer, seemingly, has obtained in some manner a remission of a condition that, medically speaking, is incurable. All your scientific training may well revolt at the thought of a remission via a person with no medical training at all who probably does not know a scapula from a spatula. I can well appreciate that your reaction as a doctor might be 'spontaneous remission' or 'wrong diagnosis'.

Now look at the situation from the healer's viewpoint. A patient who has, say, arthritis, is better. The fingers that were locked can now move and be flexed, deposits of calcium have been dispersed. Your patient's doctor, when confronted by the undeniable evidence, may say, 'Good, I am so pleased for you; sometimes these things happen'.

It may surprise you to know that the majority of your patients will not tell their doctors that they have been to consult a healer unless a direct question is put to them on the lines of, 'How did this happen?'

You may feel that your efforts are not recognised by the doctor. If so, take care. It is at this point that hubris can creep in. Remember, and *never* forget, it is not *you* who have cured the patient, if cure it be. Any healing passes *through* you. You may have contributed to the cure; doubtless you have, but it is not *your* cure. If you feel unable to accept this, you may have contracted the 'Jesus Christ' syndrome. This may be cured by a walk on water.

Apart from this, no one fully knows what part the patient's self-healing process plays in a remission.

I have found that a modest approach, should you talk to doctors, can result in a tolerant attitude, although this may range from utter scepticism to acceptance of you as some sort of unqualified medical auxiliary. The most common attitude, when relations can be established, is that you are thought of as a lay psychotherapist. As far as I am concerned, that's fine. My one real concern is that my patient gets better. That I play some part in the process is reward enough. I do not care who cures whom.

I have had doctors as patients. I have been called in by doctors to help and in certain cases had patients referred to me by them. I always make the point in these situations that I am serving in an auxiliary role and that the doctor has sole charge of the case.

This is only right; it is the doctor who may have to sign the death certificate, not me.

As I was preparing the notes for this chapter I came across a letter sent to me by a doctor who had asked me to attend a patient of his with advanced cancer. The patient, Tom, died. But, after his passing, the doctor concerned (whose name I shall not mention for professional reasons although the letter is available for inspection by any serious researcher, providing confidentiality is observed) sent me the following letter:

> Dear Mr Butler
> Thank you for all your efforts with TW. We were clearly both on a losing wicket. However, I am sure you were able to help him through those last few weeks and I am certain he did not suffer as much pain as previously.

You may think it odd that I include a letter where the patient did not get better. Not at all. One of the most important functions a healer can perform is to help someone over from this side of life to the other when it is their time to depart.

In the UK, an enormous amount of good work is being done by the Confederation of Healing Organisations in co-operating in clinical experiments with healers and the medical profession in an effort to evaluate objectively the work of healers under test conditions. The CHO are also seeking to obtain recognition for healers and establish the status of healing as a therapy. You may think this is rather obvious, but do keep in mind that the UK is fortunate in that there are few restrictions on healing. In the United States, there is a government-appointed agency, the National Institute of Health (NIH) Office of Alternative Medicine (OAM), which was created to identify and evaluate unconventional health care practices. In some other countries healing is against the law and healers can be prosecuted for breaking the law. That is why you can get healers from other countries who call themselves 'The Reverend ...', not because they claim any special religious zeal (although some do), but to avoid prosecution.

I have every sympathy with the aims and work of the CHO. It is only fitting that their work, currently under the chairmanship of Denis Haviland, CB, MA, should be better known. For example, prior to the issue of the code of conduct which is now in force, the CHO circulated the provisional version to those who could be considered interested parties. I list extracts from Appendix D of the CHO circular dated 5 November 1988:

The British Medical Association requested one amendment which we have now incorporated in the Code.

The Royal College of Nurses support the use of complementary medicine and, subject to confirmation after wider consultation, regard the Code as acceptable.

The Royal College of Midwives have proposed an amendment to the Code which has been accepted.

The Royal College of Physicians welcomed the Code and said: 'It appears to be very detailed and comprehensive as does the list of functions and objectives of the Confederation.'

The Royal College of General Practitioners said: 'The College very much welcomes the intentions of the Confederation in drawing up the Code of Conduct. We endorse the need for appropriate control and welcome the safeguards which are suggested in relation to the medical profession. We hope very much that these comments will be helpful to you.'

A spokesman for the Royal College of Surgeons said: 'The developments that you described are interesting and the statement on medical policy and ethics and the Code of Conduct have clearly been prepared with great care. I do not see any need for amendment of the latter. The College will be very interested to hear the results of the clinical trials which are being instituted.

'I am grateful to you for drawing the attention of the College to your worthy objectives and proposals and I wish you every success in their implementation.'

Sir James Watt, then President of the Royal Society of Medicine, commenting on the reorganisation of the CHO as a whole, said, 'This is highly encouraging for it does reflect on the energy and percipience you have shown to bring the standards and qualifications of the organisations to a degree which would now be considered favourable by the profession.'

Sir Donald Acheson, Chief Medical Officer of the Department of Health (speaking of AIDS patients), said: 'I am certain, despite some scepticism in some quarters, of the benefit of "healing", that any psycho-social therapy particularly involving touch would be of great benefit to this group of patients.'

I only wish that Harry Edwards and Gordon Turner were still alive to see this day when healing is being accepted as a therapy by the highest medical authorities in the land. Let us not forget the debt we owe these pioneering healers who fought for recognition from the medical authorities.

There is a price to pay. In Great Britain the healer who is a member of an organisation belonging to the CHO, or a healer of an association which is a member of the CHO, has to undertake to conform to the Code of Conduct laid down. For healers operating in countries that do not possess such guidelines, its content could be universally adopted as a basis for particular national or state requirements. The use of such a code is not only to establish an agreement on the ethics, but is evidence of a recognition that healing is part of total health care and can be used in co-operation with the medical profession. The Confederation of Healing Organisations has laid down a full code of conduct which I find quite acceptable. By kind permission of Denis Haviland, CB, MA, Chairman of the CHO, the official Code of Conduct is reproduced on pages 137–45.

Healers tend to be individualistic people. Some object to what they see as restrictions placed on their actions, and can have strong feelings on the subject.

Gordon Turner, in *A Time to Heal*, relates the talk at a meeting where the choice of title for what was to be the National Federation of Spiritual Healers was under discussion. 'John Britnell, a co-founder, favoured the name British Association of Spiritual Healers. I pointed out that the initials spelt BASH. Had I known of the wrangles which were to occur in succeeding years I might have thought this not inappropriate.'

Then there is another view to consider. Some healers feel strongly that healing is a gift from God and, as such, cannot be taught. While I can certainly respect this stance and, indeed, have no wish to argue with the religious beliefs of anyone, there is a need to follow a code if healing is to be accepted as a serious therapy. That one has to conform may be difficult for some to accept, but there are situations where compromise should be made and a pragmatic view taken.

Some control on the activities of complementary practitioners will be introduced. I would certainly advise any would-be healers to seek membership of an association or organisation which can give them the protection that will be needed in times to come. In return, acceptance and status can be expected.

So there you have it. As far as healers in general are concerned, it is, I think, essential that you become a member of a recognised healing association or federation.

Practical aspects of healing

You have, up to now as a probationer, had to follow what your trainer has suggested. You may have had more than one trainer, or sponsor, as I prefer to term the person helping you through your apprenticeship. Let us take it that you are now ready to undertake healing on your own. You may even be given a certificate to frame and put up on your wall proclaiming that *you* are a healer.

At this point you are ready to go solo; many experienced healers will, I hope, still be ready to help you. But you cannot expect the detailed help and instruction that you have had up to now; indeed, your sponsor may well be taking on another probationer.

The first thing you have to decide is whether you want to heal as part of a team or be on your own. If you decide to be part of a group, then this is dealt with in some detail in the next chapter.

Healing on your own can be daunting at first but, to me, it is the only way that you can develop your full potential.

Your main problem may be to find a room to use for healing. If this is in your own house, you will need the support of your family. You will need a room you can call your consulting room. I have always been fortunate in this respect, having had a study which has doubled as a consulting room. Some healers keep a special room – even if it is a small spare bedroom – as a healing sanctuary that is used for no other purpose than seeing patients. This is no bad thing, as over the years an atmosphere of peace and healing builds up. This is often felt by a patient when coming into the room. A new young patient came to see me and remarked as he entered my study, 'Great vibes'. At least, that is what I think he said.

Whatever room you use, it is essential it be inviting, the sort of room where you would feel quite at ease when entering. In winter, do make sure that your room is warm; it is not conducive to healing to enter a cold, bleak room.

While for the initial interview I suggest that your patient be seated in a comfortable chair, you will find seating them on a stool most helpful when you are healing as you can then move round the patient should you need to do so. In your room you will also need an additional chair to accommodate any relative or friend of your patient who may be there too.

The initial interview with your patient is important. I have known a first session last over three hours. However, this was in the case of a woman who had been advised to have a breast removed owing to cancer. It depends on the individual case as to the length of time you take, and whether you wish to deal only with the symptom (for example a migraine pain), or whether you want to help the patient find the possible cause of the problem. I do appreciate that there will be circumstances when you may be quite content just to remove any pain or discomfort that your patient is experiencing. Fine. It may be asking rather much of you at this stage to probe further. Indeed, some people by their nature are not well suited to this type of depth healing. It is quite arguable that a healer should not be called on to do more than pass through a power that can alleviate the distress of the patient.

But first things first. It is essential that you start by writing down information about your patient. Before you ask any questions at all, stress that any information will be kept in the strictest confidence and will not be given to any third party without the permission of your patient. A record card must be kept for each patient and each visit recorded on the card. It may be that the association or federation to which you belong specifies a certain format; if not, I suggest the following which I have used successfully for a number of years:

Name (in full) . . . . Tel. no . . . .

Date of birth . . . . Doctor . . . .

Address . . . .

. . . . Postcode . . . .

Symptoms/condition as stated by patient . . . .

. . . .

Medical diagnosis/prognosis given by patient's GP . . . .

. . . .

Previous history of illness . . . .

Any undue stress conditions . . . .

In the case of a patient who is legally under age, the parent or guardian must be with the patient. In addition, remember it is vital to obtain written consent when treating a child. Below I repeat a copy of the form used by healers of the British Alliance of Healing Associations:

I have been warned by . . . . (name of healer) that according to law I should consult a doctor concerning the health of my child . . . . (name of child)

Signed . . . . (parent/guardian)

Signature of person witnessing . . . .

In the case of an adult who has not seen a doctor and comes to you as a new patient, they should be advised to seek medical help. If it is not the intention of your patient to seek medical advice, then for your own protection ask that the following form be completed:

I have been advised that I should seek qualified medical help for myself.

Signed . . . . Date . . . .

Signature of person witnessing . . . .

Do keep these declarations safe with your notes on the patient.

I keep my notes of the first interview on a notepad and subsequently transfer such information as I need to the patient's record card. This allows me to have far more detailed notes on a patient should the condition be justified. What is vital is that each visit must be recorded.

As a matter of policy when treating patients of the opposite sex (unless I know them well), either I ask that they bring a friend with them or I ensure that a student healer of the same sex as the patient is with me. If I am healing at my own home, then I let my wife know that a patient is coming so that she is within call if required. I have never had a misunderstanding with a woman patient, but my advice is that it is best to take sensible precautions.

Before I even start writing down the name and address of a new patient, I stress that anything said to me will be kept in the strictest confidence. Furthermore, I indicate that no information will be given to a third party without the express permission of the patient.

To practise healing in depth, the healer has one real advantage over the doctor, the matter of time. The typical doctor is overworked owing to the per capita system whereby payment is made according to the number of patients registered rather than the time spent with each one. Even with the best will in the world it is difficult for a doctor, unless there are only a few patients to see, to devote more than about ten minutes to each patient. If more time is given to a patient, then a backlog builds up, and the doctor feels under even more pressure.

I must re-emphasise the need to probe gently to see if your patient has undergone any stress or trauma which might account for their condition. It is widely accepted that unpleasant life events such as the death of one's spouse or of a family member, marital separation, divorce, injury and illness will cause mental and emotional stress. What is possibly more interesting is that potentially happy events, such as marriage, marital reconciliation, holidays, retirement and Christmas, may also generate stress. Perhaps anything outside the normal pattern of our routine daily lives can upset us. This is important if you accept that between 60 and 80 per cent of illness is psychosomatic. Dr Ian Pearce's account of his treatment of Bob in the previous chapter (see pages 49–51) illustrates a typical case of psychosomatic illness.

Now you have the basic information about your patient, it is time to start healing. Yes, I know that you have probably been healing since the moment your patient came through the door, but this is the point at which your patient will expect some visible sign that healing is taking place.

The actual basics of healing have been given in Chapter 2. You will now be able to attune quite quickly, probably in a matter of seconds rather than minutes. Be positive and confident but *do not promise a cure.*

I cannot stress enough or too strongly that it is cruel to state that the patient's condition *will* be cured when you have no means of knowing if this will be so. It is quite another matter to mention that the condition your patient is suffering from has been successfully treated by healing and that remissions have been achieved; even when a complete recovery has not been possible, an easing of discomfort is quite frequently obtained.

No healer that I have ever met has had 100 per cent success with every patient. My own record is about 35 per cent remissions, 35 per cent betterment of condition to varying degrees, and 30 per cent where there is no apparent improvement.

I have heard it said by a healer to a patient, 'Healing will cure you. If you do not get better it means that you are not absorbing the healing power.' I am pleased to say this was many years ago, but think of the effect on the poor patient. Where there is no improvement the patient may well feel it is their own fault, thus lowering self-respect and increasing the mental pressure and stress.

Remember to ask your patient if any reaction is felt to your healing. I tend to sense the degree of heat in my hands that indicates to me that healing is taking place and at what level this is occurring. This is something that only experience can give you, and even with considerable experience some healers feel a limited reaction.

Do not allow your attunement to develop into a trance-like state while you are trying to introduce an alpha condition to your patient. Be fully aware at all times of where you are and what you are doing.

After you feel you have done all you can, or wish to, do at this stage, ask your patient to leave the stool and to return to sit on the chair.

Give your patient a minute or two to settle and ask, 'How do you feel?' Make a note of the response. At this point I suggest you make another appointment for your client if you feel one is required, and if the patient wants to return. Allow at least a week between visits.

Before my patient leaves, I hand over a copy of 'A Second Chance' and suggest that the sequence is followed. Even if your patient's condition is not due to a psychosomatic cause – and remember that this will be so for 60–80 per cent of cases – working through the sequence will help most people.

The other item that I give to patients is a copy of my local healers' association leaflet, which is based on that of the British Alliance of Healing Associations. The contents of this leaflet are reproduced below. Other associations and healing organisations have similar leaflets. You may think that the advice given and comments made are rather obvious, but to many people a visit to a healer is an unknown venture and, certainly in my experience, the majority of patients appreciate being given the information it contains.

Advice to patients who receive healing

What is healing?

Put very simply, healing consists of linking up the natural healing power within the body with the universal healing force which sustains us all. The healer is the link. By attuning to both the sufferer and the healing force, the healer serves as the channel through which the energies flow.

What is its purpose?
The purpose of healing goes beyond securing physical improvement. Its aim is to bring into harmony spirit, mind and body, so that you may lead a full, healthy and happy life, and possess a deeper awareness.

How long should I carry on with healing?
Sometimes healing is successful in one treatment. Far more often it is progressive: the results appear gradually. Please do not get discouraged and give up in the early stages. It is rare for anyone to continue to receive healing over a period without obtaining some benefit.

How can I help?
We do need your co-operation. Here are some of the ways whereby you can make a positive contribution:

1   Have healing regularly.

2   Have an open, expectant mind. Do not become over-anxious for early results. Wait patiently and with confidence for them to appear.

3   Realise that, very often, health or illness depends on the mind. Your thoughts can either help or hinder the smooth working of your body. If you have any old grievances, guilt complexes, resentments, fears or other harmful emotions, they can well be the cause of ill health. Try to get rid of them. Forgive those who have upset you. Accept your circumstances without resentment. If you have problems of this nature, discuss them with your healer.

4   Practise self-healing. Try always to picture yourself as fit and well. Once or twice a day, sit down quietly and visualise healing power entering the whole of your body. Several times a day, tell yourself that you are feeling better. This will help to bring about the positive frame of mind that is essential for good health.

What are we trying to achieve?
At the end of your healing, we want to see you not only physically well, but living in peace and harmony with yourself.

What about my doctor?

Healing is not intended to be a substitute for orthodox medical treatment. You should continue to consult your doctor. If you say that you are having healing, explain that its purpose is simply to stimulate the natural healing forces of the body. It does not in any way interfere with medical treatment.

What do I do when I wish to stop visiting the healer?

Obviously you do not want healing for ever, but when you decide to stop, please tell your healer. This is not just a matter of common courtesy. Healers develop a real concern for their patients and they like to know whether the healing has been successful or if there are any problems that can perhaps be sorted out. A note of thanks to your healer is always welcome.

Success and failure

I usually make a point of seeing patients three times before deciding if they would obtain greater benefit from another healer. So that the patient does not feel rejected, I use the analogy of the radio receiver that can only pick up AM or FM signals. I explain that if the patient is on AM/FM and I am transmitting on a long-wave frequency, then I cannot get through. I then try to suggest a healer who I feel may be able to help. The choice of such a fellow healer is obtained by experience; I find certain folk can heal people I am unable to help and vice versa.

You will have your successes. You will have your disappointments. The vital thing is to remain objective; only in this way can you perform to the best of your ability. Do not become emotionally involved with your patients; worrying and trying to take some of their burden will not help either of you, and will reduce your efficacy as a healer.

Be tolerant with people who are sceptical. Often the patients who benefit most are those who are brought to you by their nearest and dearest with some reluctance. On the other hand, those who come with the light of faith shining from their eyes do not always improve.

There are many healers who will tell you that they have no

need to talk to the patient in any depth. One healer in Scotland told me that he felt he just had to tap the heads of the patients as they walked in the door and they would obtain all the healing that he could give. In truth I have to say that this gentleman was a successful healer.

But I suggest to you that your remission rate will increase if you take the trouble and time to back up your healing with positive help to patients so that they can identify what may well be the source of their disease.

I want now to turn to special situations that you may encounter.

Healing children

When a child is brought to you, you cannot probe deeply to ascertain possible psychosomatic causes. But remember that young minds, uncluttered with preconceptions, are frequently more responsive to healing than the more sophisticated adult. Be gentle and suggest to the child that you are there to soothe away the pain. Often quite dramatic results can be obtained. Do not be patronising, and treat the child as a young adult. Stress that healing is a natural function and that all they have to do is to soak up the healing which will help them. If the child has not seen a doctor, you *must* obtain a consent form from the parent *before* you start healing.

Healing animals

Some healers are successful with animals. My experience is limited. I was asked by someone who had heard I was a healer to come and heal one of her horses. I must say that I tend to regard horses as dangerous at both ends and uncomfortable in the middle. I prefer my aged Volvo as a means of transport. Notwithstanding, I allowed myself to be taken to the horse. It was not in a good mood when I arrived but let me approach it and I gave healing.

Now Gordon Turner was a healer who had an affinity with animals. But even he had his problems. I quote from *A Time to Heal* (see page 154).

... I received a telegram which read: 'Come at once, dog seriously ill.' (When Gordon got there he was met by two ladies who said) 'We don't really know what's wrong, poor Scabbard won't let anyone into the room. The vet thinks he's gone mad. He has asked us to consider having Scabbard shot. It might be possible for someone to do it from the window.'

I followed them upstairs. We walked along a corridor with doors on either side. From every room came excited barking. They sounded like big dogs.

'What sort of dog is Scabbard?' I asked with a rather dry throat.

'An Alsatian. We breed Alsatians, you know. The dogs below are just pets. Our real interest is Alsatians; Scabbard is a champion. One of the best dogs we've ever bred.'

We stopped outside a door from beyond which came furious growling and rumbling. They looked at me admiringly.

'He's in there,' one of them said.

'It must be wonderful to be so trusted by animals,' added the other.

I felt trapped. On the one hand I lacked the courage to turn and flee along the corridor and on the other, the prospect of pushing the door and loosing the creature making such dreadful sounds appalled me.

They were still smiling and nodding happily. There was no escape. I grabbed the handle and pushed the door. As it opened inwards there was a positive roar from within as the dog sprang and pushed it mercifully shut.

'The poor chap seems a little cross,' I said fatuously.

'Perhaps if you went in with him?' one of the ladies remarked. At that moment I took a positive dislike to her. I took a deep breath and quickly stepped into the room. One of the ladies thoughtfully closed the door behind me.

Scabbard was huge. His size was exaggerated by the way in which every hair on his body was standing on end. He was crouched as if about to spring; his bared teeth looked as big as a piano keyboard. I closed my eyes and waited for the end. I opened my eyes. Scabbard had not moved, but I noticed he was shaking almost as much as I was. Cautiously I moved a few inches. The Alsatian gathered itself for the attack. I froze. There could be no doubt that he really meant it. Because there was no other course of action I decided to wait it out.

It must have been about thirty minutes before Scabbard moved. I realised that all was far from well with the animal. I knew it had been forty-eight hours since anyone had been able to give it food or water. But it was more than that which was wrong with the dog.

I felt the hot breath of the dog on my hand. I kept perfectly still. Something rubbed against my knee. I gave no sign that I had noticed. There was a tiny whimper and a warm tongue touched my hand.

From that point it was easy. I filled the water bowl from a wash hand basin in the room and Scabbard drank greedily, asking for more when it was empty.

Gordon goes on to tell us that Scabbard lived for another six years after his recovery and won several much-coveted awards.

After an interview on a radio programme, Gordon had a letter from a lady, Daphne Boden. She enclosed a picture of Shadow, her grey Arab mare. I quote again from Gordon's book:

Shadow had a torn Achilles tendon. She had been operated on by a brilliant surgeon at Newmarket, after which she had been put out to grass for three months.

She was still very lame and had, in the meantime, developed brucellosis and her wind was going. All in all, the situation looked very black.

The following Sunday, Daphne and her mother picked me up and drove me out to Richmond where Shadow was stabled. On the way they warned me that she was a spirited pony who did not take kindly to strangers pulling her about.

At the age of twenty-one, Shadow had turned as white as snow. She looked like an angel, and that is the way she behaved that morning. I treated her and suggested that for the next fortnight she be walked every day with someone leading her. At the end of this time I would see her again. I said that I hoped she would be completely well in a month.

On the next visit she was so much better that she could be ridden, and within a month she was absolutely sound in wind and limb.

A couple of years later I had dinner with the surgeon who had carried out the operation.

'I'll tell you what I did if you tell me what you did.'

'Sorry,' I said. 'I wish I could, but I just don't know.'

Daphne turned out to be a concert harpist and it was not long before I went to one of her recitals. She played beautifully. I sat entranced. She seemed so small beside her big concert harp.

Eventually we decided that we would like to get married. It happened so suddenly that it surprised everyone, including Daphne and me.

One of the first people we told was Shadow, but she was not in the least surprised. She had planned it that way all the time.

I am sorry to say that Gordon Turner died at the age of 50 after less than four years of marriage. He was a great man who did a great deal for healing. I have always held him in the highest regard and would like to think that the extracts from his book are a small tribute to his memory. In his obituary in *Psychic News* it was reported, 'Gordon loved animals and was responsible for curing many of them. Despite treating a wide variety, including a bear and an otter, never once was he bitten or scratched.'

Healing in the garden

Those of you who are keen gardeners can often use healing to advantage. Plants respond to healing as does every other living thing.

The old concept of 'green fingers' or a 'green thumb' is healing ability combined with empathy and love for the plants. My late mother-in-law, Mary Wardrop, possessed this ability developed to a fine art. Anything she touched grew with the love that she gave. I recall a tour of Scotland after which certain species of plants which she had obtained as cuttings sprang up in her garden. She had a remarkable touch.

People will scoff at this sort of talk as old country folk tales. Not so. This is not speculative but based on scientific fact. For those who may care to research further I would refer them to the work of Professor N Smith at Rosary Hill College, Buffalo, USA. She asked a well-known healer, Col Estabany, to undertake a series of experiments which were highly successful. A series of tests was also undertaken by Dr Bernard Grad at the Allen

Memorial Institute, McGill University, Montreal, with Col Estabany, where the results were subject to strict double-blind controls (source B Grad, 'A Telekinetic Effect on Plant Growth', *International Journal of Parapsychology*, Vol. 5, spring 1963, pages 117–33). There are scores of other reports that you can research if you have that sort of mind. For me the test on the two bulbs given at the end of Chapter 1 is enough ...

On a more practical level I recall the tale – where I heard it or read it I cannot remember – of the old countryman who had a beautiful garden. It was his pride and joy. He was retired and spent as much time as he could tending the plants and flowers he loved. The local vicar came by one day while old Jack was working away.

'You know, Jack, when I see all this beauty I marvel at the wonders of God!'

To which Jack replied: 'Aye, vicar, but you should have seen the mess it was in before I gave Him some help.'

Test your progress 4

After you have been healing on your own for six months, write to the patients whom you have treated and not heard from since, asking how they are and if they have benefited from healing.

This is not an ego trip for you to receive letters of gratitude. It is an attempt by you to:

1   Obtain statistical information as to your success rate.

2   Consider those cases where your patient did not obtain benefit. In these cases ask yourself:

> a) Was there anything else I should or could have done to help this person?
>
> b) Is there something else that other healers do which gives them a higher success rate?

In another six months do the project again, excluding the patients to whom you have already written, and compare the results of the two groups.

5

Healing with Others

You may not be able or indeed wish to heal from your home. In this case, a healing group or centre may be the only alternative unless you are prepared to rent or borrow a room for healing.

Some healers make house calls, visiting their patients in their homes. If someone cannot come to see me for healing, I prefer to send distant, or absent, healing. This technique is described in Chapter 7.

Having said that, many healers, often husband and wife teams, or healing partnerships of perhaps a healer and probationer, would rather heal at the patient's home in preference to having them visit the home of the healer. I know of two healers who travel long distances to visit patients. It boils down to a personal choice of what suits you, but there is an alternative: the healing group.

Organising a healing group

At a healing group or centre, you co-operate with fellow healers, rather like doctors in a group practice. I shall detail the advantages and disadvantages of this method later in the chapter, but first let me give you the basic guidelines of how such a group should be run.

The first requirement is a venue. I have found that the choice of meeting place is an important factor. A stark community centre is not always the best selection. Perhaps one of your group is prepared to offer their own house, or some rooms as a centre; more frequently, it is advisable to hire a hall or rooms. My own group was fortunate in that we were able to hire the local Friends Meeting House for our healing group. In addition to a hall, we were able to use several rooms and alcoves. I have found that the Society of Friends, Quakers as most people call them, are most co-operative in making their premises available at a nominal rent to groups who have an altruistic aim. You will also find that Unitarian Churches are often quite receptive to their halls being used for healing.

At any healing group or centre, it is essential to have some basic organisation, otherwise, with the best will in the world, a degree of chaos will show itself. There has to be a leader, someone in charge who is prepared to say 'the buck stops here'. When I ran such a group in Leicester, about 16 years ago, I found it essential to establish a procedure which all the members of the group followed; mine worked like this:

1   A receptionist was appointed. In our case we were fortunate in having a nurse from the local hospital who had received benefit from healing and wanted to pay something back. However, the receptionist could be a healer, a probationer with some experience, or a friend of healing.

Such a person may be someone who wants to help but appreciates their healing gift is not ready for development at this time. It is essential that the receptionist – greeter, perhaps, may be a better title – should be pleasant in manner and have the ability to put people at their ease. Remember that this is a most vital link in the chain. The first impressions that prospective patients obtain depend in no small part on the reception they receive when coming to the centre. The receptionist will be the first link, the first contact that the patient will have with healing. The impression made must be of caring concern.

In Britain the receptionist must ensure that the appropriate records and forms are completed in accordance with the Code of Conduct. In addition, I would draw your attention to my comments on the need to keep accurate records which I have detailed in the previous chapter (see pages 66–8).

2   After the documentation has been completed, the patient's records should be passed to the group leader who will decide which healer will deal with the case.

3   The healer assigned to the patient, probably with one or more probationers to assist and observe, will then undertake the attunement and treatment.

It could happen that the healer first treating the patient is unable to attune and feels, perhaps, it is better that another healer takes over. In this event, the group leader is notified and another healer is asked to undertake the healing.

4   There is often a tendency for patients, after treatment, to want to hang around. It is best for the healer to refer the patient back to the reception desk when healing has been completed, with a suggestion that a further appointment be made in a week's time if the healer thinks this is justified.

5   I would remind you that the notes on the patient you have just treated should always be written up before dealing with the next patient.

That is how it should work. Sometimes it does. The temptation is to turn the centre into a communal gathering when, after treatment, patients are given tea or coffee with, perhaps, a biscuit or home-baked bun. A pleasant chat is then had by all. If that's what you want, fine. My own feeling is that, if the atmosphere is one of a clinic rather than a social evening, not only will the healers be able to get on with their work but the patient will value the time spent with the healer. There is an old adage in the trade, 'Never know your healer too well'.

I fully appreciate that there is a need for many people to talk through their feelings and problems in the way I have described in the previous chapter. I suggest that this need can best be met by having a healing counsellor or helper. The function of such a helper is to listen to what the patient wishes to talk about.

In this respect I would like to quote from a book review I wrote for *Healing Review*, the magazine of the National Federation of Spiritual Healers, No. 23, autumn 1985, when dealing with Pat Young's book, *Nursing the Aged*. Pat included a chapter by Alison Charles-Edwards, a former ward sister on a terminal care ward, which shows her empathy when she discusses emotional support. Alison comments: 'Half an hour sitting with patients, sharing their fears, is a much better use of time than serving up unlimited cups of tea.'

As in any group, be it a church council or a political meeting, all is not always sweetness and light, however worthy the cause or aims. You and I are but human beings, as are our fellow healers.

We are therefore all prone to the same pettiness, jealousies and feelings as everyone else. Just because we are healers, you and I cannot assume we are immune; in fact it is quite possible that, owing to increased sensitivity, healers are more likely to be quite touchy, particularly if their methods of healing are brought into question.

The leader of the group has to maintain a careful balance to ensure harmony at a healing centre, especially if strong personalities try to assert themselves unduly.

Another problem which can face a group practice is that of lack of patients. One would expect, if no charge is being made and some remissions have been obtained, that a large queue would form before the doors open. That has not been my experience. I have known four healers, three probationers, a receptionist and a counsellor wait half an hour for the first patient to turn up! Then, over a two-hour period, only three patients attended. The healers looked as if they were in a queue for patients.

Publicity

With a new group practice, it is advisable to obtain some publicity, be it a postcard in the window of the local health food shop or a notice in the local paper. Sometimes it can help to interest your local radio station or newspaper in the fact that a new healing centre is opening. If this course is taken, be careful about making any claims for betterment that you cannot substantiate, and even those that you can. The vast majority of reporters are honest, hard-working folk but, as in all professions, there are one or two not above distortion for the sake of a good story. Remember that most reporters will try to make a story interesting and, in doing so, may well highlight the spectacular remissions, which is, of course, fair comment. What is not so nice is what happened to Gordon Turner.

Gordon relates an incident in *A Time to Heal*. At the time, he was working as resident healer at the Spiritualist Association of Great Britain headquarters in London. A reporter from a popular Sunday newspaper asked him for an interview. Gordon gave one, but explained that he was so overworked he could not cope with anything further.

> 'Can you cure cancer?' I answered this cautiously. 'There are people still living who came to me with terminal cancer as long as fifteen years ago.' They printed a two-page centre spread with plenty of photographs. It stated categorically that I claimed to cure cancer. The result was catastrophic!
>
> At my clinic people fought past my receptionist and pushed their way into my consulting room. Letters poured in by the thousand.
>
> One night I was opening these letters in my room in London when the whole weight of it hit me. So many of them were from helpless, lost people. 'I have cancer of the throat and the doctor says ...'; '... my baby has leukaemia ...'; 'My husband has ...'; and always: '... please heal him ...'; 'please heal me.'

Gordon's own health suffered from the burden that was laid upon him. In retrospect it might be said that the situation could have been dealt with by a planned response but Gordon, at the time, was already overextended even before the article came out.

So publicity for your healing centre can be helpful, but if overhyped it may prove counter-productive.

Assuming that all goes well and you have a steady flow of patients, the probability is that numbers will increase if the results are satisfactory. I have always thought that you should not try to market healing. Your best publicity is always personal recommendation from patients who have benefited from healing. Not all healers will agree with this view. I have known some who will approach people in a direct way if they know a person is ill, announce that they are healers and then proffer their services. A good healer should not have to tout for patients.

Problem patients

Another problem that all healers face and which healing centres seem to attract, is that of the permanent patient. I do not mean the obviously hypochondriac, but the patient who has, say, arthritis, has obtained maybe 60 per cent improvement but is looking for the other 40 per cent to give a total remission. Unless you are careful, this type of patient will turn up each week with a trusting smile saying, 'Now the worst is over, perhaps the rest will go.' A few weeks further on and the tune may change to, 'Well, if I'm not getting any better, we're still keeping it at bay.' If you feel no more can be done, you should say so.

Maybe you cannot bring yourself to say in such a direct manner that there is no more that you think can be done. In this case, the gentle way is to say to the patient that a visit once a month is enough instead of every week, then, after a couple of months, say once every three months. My own view is that it is better to discharge the patient saying, 'If the condition worsens again, come back and see us.'

One healer told me while I was writing this book that he had seen a patient 247 times over a four-year period. I am afraid I do not have this degree of dedication. But, as always in healing, you must act as you feel is correct for you.

With the permanent patient, do not be tempted to hand the case over to a probationer; it is unfair to give a pupil a 'no hope' case. As I type this, I am sure that a fellow healer somewhere will read the previous sentence and think, 'Ah, but that's just what I did, and the patient *did* get better.' Maybe so; one thing about healing is there are always surprises waiting for you.

Advantages of group healing

There are certain definite advantages to a group healing centre. These are as follows:

1 You have a commitment to a given period of time only once or twice each week.

2 You do not need to have people in your home if your domestic arrangements are not conducive to healing.

3 Should you be inexperienced or unsure of yourself, a centre allows you to refer to a more experienced healer should you wish to do so.

4 Some healers are better with some illnesses and conditions than others. Strange, but true. It may well be that you have a high success rate with, say, back problems. On the other hand, a fellow healer at the centre may be obtaining good results when treating arthritic patients. A healing centre enables you to refer patients to a colleague.

5 You will recall that I mentioned in the previous chapter the way that some healers are able to attune to certain patients but not others. When you are part of a healing group, it is a simple matter to suggest that, if you are unable to attune, your patient should transfer to another healer who may well be just across the room.

6 The record-keeping can be centralised so that, should you be unable to attend one session, a fellow healer can deal with a patient who normally sees you.

Drawbacks of group healing

There are also disadvantages, such as:

1 Some healers and patients prefer the more intimate atmosphere of the healer's home rather than the slightly clinical feeling generated in some healing centres.

2 At home you can heal in whatever way you wish – providing, if you are practising in the UK, you act within the Code of Conduct – and at those hours and on such days as suit you.

3 Should you, by nature, be a loner, then you might find it difficult and inhibiting to work with others and to have to conform to those standards laid down by the group leader.

In the end it all comes down to a matter of personal choice and circumstances. There is a compromise: some healers I know attend a healing group once a week but see additional patients at home.

I look forward to a time when more health centres – as opposed to sick centres – can be established offering a variety of complementary and alternative treatments at one clinic. A high degree of co-operation is needed for such projects but it is a concept well worth investment and development.

The founding and the funding of such an enterprise would be a problem, however. In the UK I cannot see the National Health Service paying for such centres, even though in the long run they might well reduce the number of people who need to attend hospitals.

Test your progress 5

At your healing group, when the last patient has gone and the evening's healing is over, ask all the members, including the receptionist and the counsellor, to sit round in a circle.

Select half of the patients that the group has on its books.

Ask the healer who has the responsibility for each particular patient to keep them in mind for extra healing.

Request all the members of the circle to attune so that a golden circle of light is in a ring around the circle. Once this is done, extend the circle so that the golden ring is in the form of a dome over the whole of the group. Then ask the group to visualise a blue healing light blending with the gold.

In turn, ask each healer to envisage their patient being led into the golden-blue dome. The healer should name the patient and project the patient's image into the healing light. Each member of the group should then give healing to the patient named.

After, say, two minutes, ask the next healer in the group to name a patient and go through the same procedure.

When half of the patients on the group's books have been covered, then close the circle.

It is vital that the *same* patients are nominated at each session during the test period.

Compare the remission rate between those patients who have received the additional group healing and those who have not. If there is a significant variation, then I suggest that as a matter of course every patient is included in the healing dome at the end of each of your healing sessions.

6

Healing as a Profession

Like Mr Punch's advice on marriage, my initial reaction to regarding healing as a profession is to say 'don't'. There are many folk who hear the call to heal and feel they have a mission. Great. Yet most healers can follow this vocation and still carry on with their everyday job, be it as a bricklayer or bus driver, supermarket cashier or attorney.

The only justification for healing full-time is that the healer is unable to see all the patients requiring healing in the spare time that is available.

I know of one part-time healer who is booked up for ten weeks ahead. I asked him whether he had thought of healing full-time and his reply was quite direct. 'I cannot heal full-time because I have a wife and three young children to support, and I do not think healing is a reliable source of income.'

In Britain there are more than 10,000 healers. Only a small proportion of these are professional. Of these, there may be those part-time healers who make a charge to every person, but do not rely on healing as their sole source of income. If you said there were 100 full-time professional healers, that would be one per cent of healers.

Healing is available from a dedicated number of people to whom the concept of healing is one of service. These folk feel that healing their fellow human beings is a privilege and they are anxious to share their gifts. Since they make no charge, or at best will accept a donation which most times is passed on, why should someone choose to go to a professional healer and pay for healing when they can have the same treatment free of charge elsewhere?

The only possible reasons are that the professional healer obtains a much higher rate of remission than the non-professional, that the professional healer has a 'name' and is well-known via the media, or that the patients feel that they must pay. The last reason may seem odd, but I can assure you that there are people who feel they must pay for everything in life. If they do not pay, often they do not get better.

If you discount any media hype, and the person who feels that payment should be made – which can be dealt with by a donation – then you have the one remaining factor, a greater rate of remission when, it does seem, the patient derives great benefit. It is a fact that some healers are more efficacious than others. Their patients have a higher rate of remissions. In consequence their services are in such demand that they cannot hope to see in their spare time all those who require healing.

Many healers who decide to become professional feel that, rather than charge set fees, they should rely on donations. Let me give you some practical evidence about this.

I know of two professional healers in the same area, one of whom charges twice as much as the other. A third charges a fraction of that cost and a local clairvoyant charges for a reading but not for healing – and gets more clairvoyant work.

In *Professional Healing – My Way* by Don Greenbank (see page 154), Don mentions his experiences. The book was sent to me for review, and, as a consequence of this, Don and I exchanged letters. He told me that when he started healing in Bradford in the 1960s, for the first four years he took home £4.00 ($7.00) a week; for the next five years he took £7.00 ($11.50) from the practice. To those of you unable to recall those days I would mention that my own salary was £105.00 ($175.00) a week plus expenses working for a major electrical company as a sales manager. I am quite sure Don had a far more responsible job than I. The following is an extract from his book:

> Let me tell you of my experiences ...: being more than naive
> when I opened my Sanctuary, my starry-eyed beliefs saw no
> flaws that the quality of my faith could not overcome. With

dependence on the charity of people's donations, my education into a mixture of people and their money was under way with a swing. Immediately you step into this new role, bang go all your pension rights and golden handshakes. You gaze at the stack of unpaid bills with the familiarity of an old friend. A time limit is set in your mind: 'I can afford to lose so much and then that's it, we close.' This time limit will come and go, and yet somehow you make out and always manage just to scrape through.

However elevated your views, thoughts and ideals are, you as a healer are still subject to the world's system of trade. Your talent is as much a gift as an artist's or writer's ...

The plaintive cry from the pseudo-religious critics is that healing is a pure gift from God and should therefore be free. They forget conveniently the very many calls on a healer's pocket, such as rent, rates, electricity, heating, telephone, postage ...

Some patients even thought I was part of the National Health Service, so they didn't feel the need to leave anything! I do remember clearly one man, who, incidentally, received a wonderful improvement. After I had treated him, he drew a huge roll of notes from his pocket, asked for some change and when that was provided placed one shilling – 5p (8 cents) – on the collection plate with the air of a second Dale Carnegie!

Then there was the man who pleaded abject poverty and left nothing; every time he came for healing he left his brand-new car round the corner.

The months of financial worries grew into years, with my pile of bills going up and down like a yo-yo. There comes a time though, when you feel that any more shabby treatment will sour your gift and therefore, very reluctantly, you have to accept the inevitable and make a fixed charge for treatment.

I met Major Bruce MacManaway at several Health and Healing courses that were run at various universities in the 1970s by the Wrekin Trust.

Bruce discovered his healing gift at Dunkirk in 1940 when, as a young army officer, he treated soldiers who were wounded and found he could help them. I would stress that Bruce was not with the Royal Army Medical Corps, but a combat soldier.

After he retired from the army, he founded a healing centre at West Bank, Fife, in Scotland. Here he treated patients from all over the world and was held in high esteem. In addition to healing, he also took pupils whom he trained as healers. The pupils paid a premium, or fee, and in return obtained the benefit of Bruce's undoubted experience.

In my talks with him at the Wrekin Trust courses, Major MacManaway always maintained that people should pay for healing if they could afford to do so. In his opinion, this established a professional relationship and enabled the healer to enjoy a reasonable standard of living.

Don Greenbank was not the only professional healer to suffer in his early days. His story is similar to several I have heard from healers who have attempted to make healing a profession. Perhaps the most graphic account is that of Gordon Turner given in *A Time to Heal* (see page 154). He talks of wealthy patients who would sometimes arrive at his sanctuary in one of the poorer parts of north London. The attitude of some of those wealthy patients was quite extraordinary. They would thank him profusely and ask about his fees:

> 'I don't charge a set fee. There's a collection plate on the hall table. You may leave what you like.'
>
> 'I say! That's wonderful. You're doing fine work. Of course I'd like to support it. Tell you what, I'll leave a really big donation at the end of my treatment.'
>
> They never did. One millionaire who was suffering from a rare malignant blood disease promised to donate a fitted carpet for the sanctuary when he was healed. After about five treatments his hospital tests were clear. The specialist had told him that his case must have been one of mistaken diagnosis. He telephoned excitedly and told me the news.
>
> 'Now, about that carpet. Can you be at home tomorrow afternoon? I'll bring the patterns round personally.'
>
> Of course he never showed up. Years later I walked into a restaurant and he was seated at the table opposite mine. Although he was only halfway through the meat course, he grabbed his coat and fled.
>
> The most blatant case of this kind I can remember was a man who arrived to see me in a bath chair. He'd arrived in a chauffeur-driven Rolls Royce and was accompanied by a manservant.
>
> 'I've been like this for two years,' he told me, 'and I've

spent a fortune trying to find a cure. I've been the length of Harley Street, to clinics in Switzerland, even Lourdes. In fact, everywhere. If you can cure me, you can name your own fee.'

I gave him the same reply I gave everyone at that time. 'There's a collection plate in the hall. Leave what you like. In any case, I can't promise to heal you.'

I gently ran my fingers down his spine. They reacted strongly to a spot near the base in the area of the fifth lumbar vertebra. I concentrated for a moment and then pressed it gently with my hand. There was a loud crack.

'Try to stand,' I told him. 'Your legs may feel weak from lack of use.'

He stood up and then took two or three paces. 'Good God! I haven't done that for two years.' As he gathered confidence, he strode up and down, sat, stood up again, touched his toes and lifted his knees up and down like a guardsman marking time.

'It's a miracle,' he told me. 'I'll never forget what you've done for me.' He left pushing his own bath chair.

My curiosity got the better of me and I followed him up the hall to see what he would leave. When he reached the plate he took out his wallet, hesitated, and put it away again. Reaching into his trousers pocket he extracted a handful of small change. He carefully selected a two-shilling piece – 10p (16 cents) – and placed it on the plate and opened the front door. He hesitated for a moment, and then returned to the plate, removed the florin and, having replaced it with a threepenny piece (1½p or about two cents), hurried out of the front door.

After the experiences of Gordon and Don can you blame a person who is healing full-time for making a reasonable charge? I am sometimes asked what is a fair amount as a fee. I doubt if there are any hard and fast rules; much depends on your overheads and what standard of living you require.

If you use a room in your own house, then you have less expense than a healer who has to hire a room or rooms. Another factor to consider is how long you will be spending with each patient. My sessions average about an hour for the first interview with a patient and half an hour on subsequent visits. Other healers find that half an hour is enough for a first visit, with perhaps 20 minutes for a repeat healing session.

Remember you may only see two or three paying patients a day. If, as a part-time healer, however busy, you start charging a fee, you may well find your patient list falling dramatically. Investigate local charges of similar practitioners and set your fees accordingly.

You will need to adjust your figures to account for the cost of living in your own area. Another factor to bear in mind is the position of pensioners or those on a restricted income. In these situations I would never refuse to treat patients because they could not afford to see me. Many healers offer reduced rates, often half their normal fee, for those short of money. In addition, a free clinic may be held at which no charge of any sort is made. This may take place, say, once a week on a first-come, first-served basis.

When fixing a scale of charges, remember that you will be a self-employed person with all the responsibilities that this will bring. You will not be able to ensure a reliable income of a fixed sum each week, month or year; there is no holiday or sick pay; there are no pension rights that go with the job, to name but a few of the difficulties you will have to face.

Remember you will have to file tax returns and therefore careful accounts will have to be kept. There are plenty of courses on basic account-keeping if you feel the need. Or there are several computer programs that can do virtually everything for you at the touch of a button – all you do is feed in the basic data.

It may seem odd to talk about such matters in a book on healing but, if you are thinking of being a professional healer, you have to establish certain basic business procedures, otherwise you could find yourself in a real muddle.

Test your progress 6

This chapter has dealt with healing as a profession.

Before you decide to embark on such a course of action, I want you *truly* to test your progress. Ask yourself:

1 Why do I want to be a professional healer?

2 Am I prepared to make sacrifices to achieve this?

3 Are those dependent on me prepared to share these sacrifices?

4 Do I have the basic stamina to undertake what is often an exhausting vocation?

5 Why can I not just heal in the evenings and at weekends?

You may feel that I am being hard-nosed on the subject. You're right.

I know I can only give healing to a certain number of patients at any one time. Were I to exceed that number, I could not give of my best. To undertake what I *know* is too much for myself would be quite unfair to all concerned, not least my patients.

7

Distant Healing

Distant healing is, of course, healing given from a distance. Absent healing is another term used to indicate that the healer is not in a face-to-face situation with the patient. Both terms mean the same thing and are interchangeable, but confusion can be caused if this is not clearly understood.

It does not matter if your patient is in the next road or halfway across the world, distant healing really can be very effective.

I do not pretend to know how distant healing works – although I give the views of several healers in a later chapter – but I do know how to make it work. The techniques are quite simple once you are experienced in basic attunement.

Practising distant healing

Attune to someone who is ill, as if they were sitting in your room. The method I use is:

1 I visualise the patient and attune so that I am ready to heal.

2 I move my hands, which I hold in front of me, palms towards each other, about 30 cm (12 in) apart and adjust them to ensure the maximum healing power is present.

3 Still maintaining my attunement, I swivel in my chair until I sense the direction of the patient. This seems to work like radar – it sounds silly when you read it, but it works.

4 When I feel maximum intensity, I envisage the patient between my hands. I then send healing in the normal way until I feel the power drop.

5 As the healing decreases, I gently break contact, my last thought being of the patient glowing with health.

The technique given above is a basic form of distant healing. However, there are other sequences and methods which can be used; if I do not seem to be obtaining a positive result, then I may combine my basic method with one or more of the following:

1   a) Visualise your patient in a sphere of light.
b) Attune to the patient and, as you do so, allow healing to be sent via yourself in the form of a beam which envelops the sphere of light with a blue and golden series of rays which are charged with healing power.
c) Allow these active rays of healing to flow through the sphere to your patient. Continue until all healing force has been absorbed, then gently break contact.

2 In cases of depression, attune to your patient and envisage a happy, laughing person who is quite carefree. If you sense a black or grey cloud of depression around your patient, then try to visualise a pulsating, lively light of golden sun breaking up the clouds and filling your patient with joy, light and laughter.

3 With malignant growths, I imagine the growth between my hands and try to shrink it. I also think of the growth being gobbled up by shoals of piranha fish who only like to eat malignant cells and refuse to consume healthy tissue.

4   If I have a case of arteriosclerosis – a thickening and rigidity of the middle coat of medium-sized arteries – I equate the condition to a furring-up of pipes in a hot water system and visualise the system being cleaned out by solvent liquid healing which breaks up the silt and flushes it away. I then envisage healing moving into the walls of the arteries so that they return to a youthful elasticity, capable of expanding as the pressure of blood increases at any one point.

I do not claim that these techniques are unique; many healers use these methods or variants of them. The basic concept of betterment is always the common factor as is attunement to your patient so that you are in an alpha state.

Let your imagination range over the variations on the basic themes and methods given above. If, for example, a person has a broken bone, envisage the bone knitting together. Should your patient have arthritis, then visualise the calcium deposits around the joints being broken up and dispersed by healing.

Distant healing now comprises most of my own healing work. Like everything else it has to be organised or you will get in a muddle. Remember that you have as much responsibility to an absent healing patient as you do to someone who comes to see you. My method of working is:

1 A request is received for healing. If it is a letter written by the patient this helps me to attune, as does a photograph.

2 I immediately place the patient on my healing list and attune to them every day.

3 I reply to the patient's letter asking for a weekly progress report and, in the case of adults, enclose a copy of 'A Second Chance' which I ask them to undertake and work through. In my letter of reply I ask that they put a few minutes aside each day to attune to me, sitting in a receptive mood.

4 The healing is maintained until a remission is reported or a weekly progress report is no longer received.

5 In the event of a report of no progress beyond a certain point, then I may well suggest the services of another healer.

I find that my results from distant healing are, as a percentage, similar to those obtained by contact healing. The only major variant is where there is a need for psychotherapy, but even here, if the patient has worked through 'A Second Chance' the results seem to equate to face-to-face healing.

As you read this you may be thinking that the total concept of absent healing is unrealistic, and it must be that the person who is asking for help just has faith in the healer. I can well understand this viewpoint, but would mention that distant healing works with children, animals and those patients – for example in an accident or who have had a stroke – who are unaware that healing has been requested.

So that you may know that distant healing works, I shall give some extracts from letters I have received from patients who have benefited from absent healing:

Bournemouth

Dear Mr Butler,
      Thank you very much for your kind letter and for putting my husband on your absent healing list. He is brighter today and a good change is apparent in his condition.

Aylestone

      ... I was amazed to read your comments on the underlying cause of my illness. Yes, there was a very miserable period in my life ten years ago ...
      You will be pleased to learn that at long last I have wakened up several mornings free from neuritis, the miserable burning pain in my thighs which has tortured me each night for ten years. I am so grateful.

Midlothian

      You were very kind and understanding with me when I wrote to you. You sent absent healing to me and effected an almost complete cure of a contracting finger in my left hand. As I am a music student (pianist), I am sure you will understand how much I appreciate your help. I have now been able to resume my studies thanks to you.

Cobham

      Last Sunday I saw Mrs W, whom I asked to be put on your healing list because she was in such pain with her back when I visited her the month previously; I would now like to add she is completely without pain, and there is no need for any further distant healing.
      Naturally she is extremely grateful and sincerely thanks you.

Leicester

Dear Pat,

... I would be grateful if you would consider undertaking an assignment for me.

Roughly 18 months ago my mother (who had no hearing in one ear for 23 years) became totally deaf. This occurred shortly after the death of her mother from carcinoma. Her physician, noting the absence of any peripheral damage to the ear, diagnosed a perceptive deafness, i.e. damage to the micro vessels of the inner ear. It appeared to me, however, that her condition and previous medical history did not conform to this diagnosis.

She was plagued by noises in her head ... My impression of her condition was not of a psychotic reaction, but a conversation hysteria. I asked a psychiatrist colleague in Scotland to see my mother, and he agreed there was a grief reaction present.

Both my mother's psychiatrist and myself have felt the only possible treatment to be time, and we expected the condition to resolve itself in due course. We have now tried a nine-month cycle of a major tranquilliser and have now prescribed an anti-depressant. Although chemotherapy helped, we feel we can do little more.

Would you please consider any way in which you and your colleagues might be able to alleviate her burden?

I replied to this by return post, saying that I would send absent healing to his mother in Scotland. Not having heard for a few weeks, I wrote again and asked him how things were going. He replied:

Dear Pat,

I must apologise for my lack of feedback during the past few weeks regarding my mother's progress. I have not been in touch with Scotland for a fortnight, but last night received a telephone call from my mother who appeared to be restored to her original condition ... Her personality and appetite have returned to a considerable extent. There is no possible explanation in terms of change of chemotherapy or other medical intervention; she attributes her improvement solely to your ministrations.

May I therefore congratulate you and your group for your efforts over the past weeks and may I exhort you to continue in your efforts with the sight of recovery on the horizon.

Many thanks Pat. I find it hard to comprehend but I cannot refute your positive intervention.

I mentioned before that distance makes no difference in the benefit that can be derived from absent healing. This is a letter I received from a patient in the USA:

Leominster, MA 01453

Dear Pat,

At the time I mailed my previous letter my infected eye started to improve and upon receiving your reply and using the 'Second Chance' further improvement has continued until there is now no infection ...

Gratefully yours

I have many other letters of this sort, but volume does not count when you consider way back in 1953 Harry Edwards published his book *The Evidence for Spiritual Healing*, wherein he listed 10,369 reports from patients who had benefited from healing. The book is 514 pages in length and contains 214,000 words.

The basic point is that distant healing works. If you are ill, it can work for you.

After I had been practising absent healing for 15 years, I was anxious to find ways whereby the success rate could be increased still further. In partnership with various groups, I tried healing circles but I still could not get the results I was seeking. Then I had the idea of a number of experienced healers working in their favourite environment at the time when they are best attuned. I called it the Hit Squad.

The Hit Squad

Whilst distant or absent healing has been used since the earliest days, during the past two years members of the Suffolk Healers Association in England have evolved a system of intensive healing.

The concept is quite simple. A number of experienced healers are encouraged to offer their services and undertake to send distant healing to a patient selected by the co-ordinator from nominations put forward from the participating healers. The patients are those with chronic conditions who have not responded to individual treatment, or those about to undergo a serious operation.

We do not meet in a group. It seems far more effective when each healer works alone. The details of the patient are passed to each healer who then concentrates on that specific patient. This is additional to each healer's normal case-load.

The results can be quite remarkable, with a clear-up rate far greater than in conventional methods – including groups of healers sending distant healing where, at the meeting, a list of patients is read out. The success rate seems to be linked to the fact that all the members of the team, in our case eight, independently send healing at the time they feel most attuned. Although the healing is sent independently, a degree of synergy applies.

One of the blessings of this system is that it allows a healer who is ill to obtain healing. The following letter is from one of our members who benefited in this way:

Lowestoft

Dear Pat,

I want to put in writing my gratitude to you and 'the team' for your help in my recent operation, which although a minor one is one that has a reputation for being at worst very painful and at best pretty uncomfortable. But also I think it is important to place on record my experience of multiple absent healing in the hope that other groups of healers who have not taken part in this activity may feel encouraged to do so.

I felt honoured some months ago to have been invited to join your 'hit squad' as you call them or 'healing commandos' as I dubbed them, and it was gratifying subsequently to hear of the successes scored in some quite difficult cases. I had already proved the efficacy of absent healing on my own with some of my own patients, but some of these results following calling up the squad in emergencies or really tough cases were truly remarkable. Now, I have to report my experience from the receiving end, and all I can say is it simply confirms what I had felt hitherto, namely that the power generated by a group of healers all working together for the named person or persons is as powerful a force for good as anything this side of the Great Kingdom I have ever been aware of. The facts of my own cases were: bi-lateral nasal polypectomy, double antrostomy and sub-mucosal diathermy – a lot of polyps to be removed, some of them big ones, the base of each antrum to be opened up (bone taken away) to allow sinus drainage, and finally cauterisation by the insertion of hot wires under the mucous lining of the nose to widen the breathing passages and lessen the chances of further polyps forming the in the future. Apparently I lost a lot of blood and was longer than usual in the recovery room for this reason, but when I came round back in the ward all I could feel was the plugging in each nostril which is always left there for 24 hours. *I felt no pain whatever, nor did I at any time afterwards.* Now, at three and a half weeks after the operation, I can breathe freely for the first time for three years and all has completely mended, painlessly.

I shall always be grateful to the 'team' for helping me to be opened to receive God's love in this way – for this, I believe, is what it is; it is difficult for us when we are very ill or under an anaesthetic to open ourselves to receive God's love (Whose healing power always goes directly to where *He* knows it is needed), but with a little outside help it *can* be done, and sometimes dramatically.

Thank you – all of you – again,

With love as ever

As I was preparing the final draft for this book, news came from Australia via the husband of a 39-year-old woman who was placed on our Hit Squad list in late 1989. She was due to have a transplant of the heart and then a transplant of a lung. After three months on the list the following report was received from Australia:

Ruth is a one-off. So her consultant physician and the entire transplant team feel. They have not experienced an improvement like hers *naturally*, in their medical experience. They had to get her off all the heavy medication she was taking when admitted, this was essential prior to a transplant operation being carried out. This procedure was pretty horrendous for Ruth and was carried out quite dramatically at the time, as her lung capacity was so poor she totally relied on pressure oxygen all the time; added to this she had heart palpitations which concerned her doctors. Then slowly she began to improve and after ten weeks was able to come off the oxygen completely, much to the amazement of the transplant team. The decision was then made, early in December, to take her off the transplant list and let nature take its course. She is on only two drugs and this, plus her positive attitude, appears to be doing the trick. Hopefully, Ruth will regain a quality of life that will be acceptable to her and that a transplant will not be necessary.

The condition that Ruth was suffering from was fibrosing alveolitis.

Test your progress 7

The test I want you to undertake now will show if you are able to pass your healing through one material to another.

Take a bottle of water, an old milk bottle will do, a watering can may be better, just as you feel. Attune and place your hands round the container as though you are passing healing energy into the water, a life force that is going to make anything that it feeds grow and grow well.

If you have a garden or greenhouse, choose a plant that may not be doing too well and needs a little help. Water it with the treated water. In other words you are not treating the plant by direct healing, but via the water you have energised.

Should you not have a garden – perhaps you live in a flat or apartment – then you can try another experiment. Buy a bunch of flowers, divide them into two groups with the same number of flowers in each. Place the flowers in two vases. Make sure you put the same amount of water in each vase, but in vase 'A' use the energised water and in vase 'B' use ordinary water. Be sure when you change the water that you energise the water for vase 'A'. Compare the length of time each vase of flowers lasts – those in the energised water should stay bright and fresh longer.

8

How Healing May Work

Nobody knows where healing comes from. The results can be seen, and the fact that some people improve as a result of treatment from a healer is beyond dispute.

In *The Reality of the Paranormal* (see page 156), Professor Emeritus Arther J Ellison, then Head of the Department of Electrical and Electronic Engineering at the City University, London, recalls a demonstration by Harry Edwards and fellow healers he watched at the Royal Festival Hall in London:

I observed a lady coming on to the stage where she revealed a large projecting goitre in her neck. One of the healers working with Harry Edwards gently stroked it for some minutes and it apparently disappeared completely. I could see quite a different silhouette against the light and a doctor with whom I discussed the matter told me that there was nowhere to which the healer could have pushed the goitre out of sight.

Of even greater interest was Harry Edwards' treatment of a number of arthritic old ladies who came up on the stage scarcely able to hobble and with their finger joints very swollen and stiff. I watched Harry Edwards place his hands against the backs of the patients and straighten them up; then he continued by manipulating their fingers. He took each finger in turn and moved it about until it seemed to be free. At the end of the process the patients appeared to be able to move their fingers in an almost natural way and left the stage walking practically normally.

I discussed this remarkable phenomenon of the apparent removal of the symptoms of arthritis with a distinguished psychiatrist. He told me that he had observed exactly the same procedure and results.

Spritual healing

There is no doubt that the one person who did more in Britain than any other to bring healing to the public eye was Harry Edwards. I do not have the space to do justice to this great man further than my comments in Chapter 1, but a biography, *Harry Edwards*, by Ray Branch has been published (see page 153). This gives you the story of this remarkable man. Harry Edwards' own book, *A Guide to the Understanding and Practice of Spiritual Healing*, published in 1950 but still in print (see page 153), clearly sets out his own views. In it he says:

> As man can direct a physical force, so it requires a spirit mind to direct a spirit force, for it belongs to the spirit realm and not to earth. So it is with the spirit healing forces, every act of healing demands independent, intelligent direction.
>
> This is easily demonstrated. With an individual healer, one witnesses healings of a widely divergent character, the restoring of an unbalanced mind, the dispersal of a growth and the correction of sight or hearing. Obviously a different quality of healing force is necessary for the three examples just mentioned.
>
> To apply the right quality of healing force in its correct strength to a given human disharmony, intelligent direction is needed. As man has never possessed this knowledge, it cannot exist within the subconscious mind ... The subconscious mind is the repository of experience. Because it has never known the way to motivate the spirit forces, the human mind cannot be responsible for the application and discrimination of these forces.
>
> We are, therefore, forced to the conclusion that the operating mind must be a spirit one; a mind that has acquired greater wisdom than man possesses.

Harry Edwards was proud to be a spiritualist, and was certain that discarnate doctors were among the healers in spirit who worked through him. The term 'spirit healer' implies, to me at least, that it is a discarnate spirit who is working through the healer. The reason I stress this point is that there is often confusion between the term 'spirit healer' and 'spiritual healer'. My own interpretation is that a spiritual healer certainly agrees that healing comes from an outside spiritual force, but not necessarily from an individual discarnate spirit. Many spiritual healers are not spiritualists. They may be of any religion.

Some spiritual healers maintain that the soul, spirit or Higher Self is healed, or activated to heal, by the outside spiritual power transferred via the healer.

God's power to heal

There are folk who called themselves 'divine healers'. They maintain that their power to heal comes directly from God and flows into the patient. I have no doubt that the majority of these healers are sincere and honest people. Just one point. If the healing comes from God, how can it fail in some cases? One 'divine' lady I asked replied, 'They don't have enough faith'.

I am reminded of the statement by Lawrence Le Shan (*From Newton to ESP*, see page 155) when he talks of psychic healing:

What was going on? The first clue came from a remark of George Bernard Shaw. He said that the shrine at Lourdes was the most blasphemous place on earth. When asked to explain his remark, he said that one only needed to look at what was there; mountains of wheelchairs, piles of crutches, 'but not a single wooden leg, glass eye or toupée!' This, said Shaw, implies a limitation to the power of God, and that *was* blasphemy.

Later in his book, Le Shan comments:

None of us do anything as well as we possibly can. Whether we are talking about climbing a rope, understanding a book, discriminating wines, or making love, we can learn to do it better. We operate far below our potential. In healing ourselves, this is also true. Although we all use our self-healing abilities (as when we cut ourselves and the body heals the cut), we use them at a level of efficiency far below their potential. In psychic healing, the situation is temporarily changed by the healer–healee interaction, so that the healee is better able to make use of his self-healing abilities. This would explain the observation of Shaw. There are no wooden legs at Lourdes because the self-healing abilities (in contrast to those of lobsters) cannot regenerate a leg. *Psychic healing can only work up to the level of self-healing abilities at their best.* All the data of the best reported cases would corroborate this hypothesis.

Le Shan makes a valid point here upon which we should ponder.

There are, and have been, masters or *avatars* who have the power to heal, regardless of the condition of the patient. The greatest of these was Jesus Christ. One living today may well be Sai Baba.

In this respect a most interesting letter was published in *Light*, the journal of the College of Psychic Studies in London, in their issue of autumn, 1978. The author was Kenneth Woodward, who I was able to contact through the good services of the then editor, Brenda Marshall. It reads:

> ... I dare to suggest that the Christian dogma of the 'forgiveness of sin' arose out of the skilled therapeutic technique of one – widely known in the West as the Master Jesus – who knew exactly when the time was ripe to persuade a 'sinner' to forgive himself; and thus how to enable him to release himself from a condition which his attachment to guilt permitted to persist. And, given the level of consciousness at that dark period of our history, He did it by *Himself,* offering the erring personality 'forgiveness'. But this He would only do on behalf of the sinner's own Spiritual Individuality.
>
> As is widely known today, many illnesses are engendered by guilt, real or imaginary. Despite the truth of this, it would be possible effectively to offer the acceptance of forgiveness only to an individual who had progressed to the point where it had become karmically possible for him to so self-accept it that it would bring about the cure of an undesirable condition, whether engendered on the mental, emotional or the physical level; or even as a result of a negative state in the soul itself. Briefly, the one who serves as 'saviour' does so by triggering off a process of 'salvation' in the 'sinner', when he has reached a state of readiness to abandon the accumulated effects of past

negative thought and action. But the 'sinner' who is about to be liberated from the effects of past deeds must have *earned* the right to it, whether he knows it or not. Thus is a 'miraculous' cure or conversion effected.

Religion of whatever school, whatever else it may offer of teaching, communion, enlightenment or guidance, cannot offer vicarious forgiveness, for this is a spiritual-psychotherapeutic technique which serves to precipitate into effect earned results by breaking through a conditioned barrier which is resistant to the manifestation of change. Forgiveness is that which each has to gain for himself through treading the path which leads to the discovery of the Self. And that path is service, in obedience to law ...

Consider the implications of Kenneth Woodward's letter. The word 'karma' is introduced, a word linked with reincarnation. Until this chapter I have deliberately kept this book secular, but I would now like to speculate a little. Who are we? What are we? What is it we are trying to heal?

My own belief is that each of us is inhabiting our physical body which is being used temporarily by our true Self, in other words our soul or *atman*, to use an Eastern term. Furthermore, when the soul leaves the body it continues its existence. In this book it is not my intention to delve into probable post-mortem states; I am not a spiritualist but I do know that life continues after the death of the body.

Healing and reincarnation

Sooner or later, your soul may well feel the need to reincarnate on Earth once again. Should a soul reincarnate, there may well be certain karmic debts that need to be repaid, and in the process some suffering, perhaps through illness or disablement, may be undertaken by the soul to achieve a state of being at one with the Infinite.

If, for example, a soul comes back to earth to travel along a certain path and is prevented from doing so by the ego's desires and longings, then the soul is frustrated. You have a desire for security and feel that this may be obtained by money. I may think that I would like a large house, fast car, a good job, etc.

What I am really doing is gratifying my ego through all things. It is not far from the thought that, 'I will be happy if I win the football pools'.

This is absurd, but if you extend the thinking beyond the obvious, then you can see the constant striving of the ego for what it thinks is happiness. Why? Because the ego is frightened. The more the material level of wealth grows, the safer the ego feels. All this enhances the ego immensely and entrenches it firmly in the body: the soul hardly gets a look in.

Now if your total self is made up of the soul, *atman*, divine spark (whichever name you care to choose), the ego (your personality), the mind (which is purely a slave to the ego in most of us) and the body, then any conflict between the ego and the soul can cause disease in the body or mind.

I would seriously suggest to you that, on occasions, the *atman*, soul or divine spark is so fed up with the way it is unable to progress that it sparks off, quite deliberately, an illness or disease in the body virtually saying, 'I have not come back here on earth to do this. I would much rather go back from whence I came and return later on and have another attempt. If this ego chooses to function without me I'll go home.'

If your soul is so imprisoned by your ego through the worry, fear and pain of your illness, it could be that your divine spark is not very bright, and perhaps it is my job, as a healer, to help fan it back into a glow if it is God's will so to do.

The type of healing I am talking about is depth healing and one must remember that healing takes place on various levels; not all healers are used for this type of work. One who was, H K Challoner, published her experiences with a most difficult and involved case, in *The Path of Healing* (see page 154). The patient was told, 'If you had not been ready to make an attempt to comply with my conditions I would not have the right, nor indeed the power, to offer to help you.'

Healing and the Higher Self

There is yet another view held by some healers. It is that the Higher Self (or the soul, or *atman*, if you prefer) of the healer is able to activate the Higher Self in the patient and, by so doing, the patient's Higher Self is able to activate their own inner healing.

Some healers dislike the word God (or Allah, Brahma, Jahweh or any other title) and prefer to talk of the universal life force. I have even been told of healers who say, 'No I am not a healer, I am a dianergic therapist.'

At this point I can sense the question, 'Who cares how a person gets better as long as he or she does?' I can go along with that some of the way, all of the way if I am to be quite objective. After all, what is a healer doing but helping people to get better? Why worry where it comes from, how and why? Well, if nothing else, it is important to the healer. Most healers feel that they are undertaking a ministry of healing, a calling to heal. Take that away and there is little motive for them to do anything at all, why should they? Without this sense of ministry or vocation, many groups and organisations would not exist.

The world would be a much sadder place without people all over the world activated by a sense of dedication.

The social services? Within limits, yes, but they can never replace the dedication of the members of so many groups who have a real calling to help people.

Consider the parable of the Good Samaritan. In the version I heard, two social workers came across the victim of a gang of robbers before the Good Samaritan arrived on the scene. They said, 'Gosh, we've got to find the guys who did this, they need help.'

Life fields and thought fields

You may have heard the terms 'L-fields' (life fields) and 'T-fields' (thought fields). They have an important part to play in our understanding of how healing may work. For a lay person to talk about scientific matters is a most hazardous undertaking. I therefore quote the basic concepts from a scientist, Dr Ian Pearce, who covers these matters in his book *The Gate of Healing* (see page 154).

> Actually, the molecules with which the body deals are, of
> necessity, so complex that they lack the stability to rest. Their

instability is such that they are forever falling apart and any device whereby they are put together again at an equivalent rate can allow the body to make use of their tremendously complex structure.

Thus we are faced with the problem of how these complex molecules can be rebuilt precisely to pattern so that each person, though composed of entirely different constituents, is immediately recognisable as the same person after an interval in which the entire body has been renewed. Moreover, we must also realise that this process of rebuilding takes place from basic materials supplied to the body in its daily food, so that the proteins and minerals of the vegetable kingdom become transformed into human flesh. Further, the body is able, when challenged, to produce entirely new substances, such as antibodies specific to a particular antigen, to protect itself against injury when required for its continuing health and existence. This extreme precision must postulate a system of control, and an understanding of this is vital to our understanding of the human creature and of the problems posed by disease and healing. Of what nature is this precise and wonderful system of control?

We owe our understanding of this process to the researches and life work of one man – the late Harold Saxton Burr – Professor Emeritus of Anatomy at the University of Yale. Burr's discovery was that all living forms, whether animal, vegetable, or of lower, less differentiated nature, are associated with electro-magnetic fields. These fields, which can be measured and mapped by modern electronic instruments, are believed by some to be the controlling mechanisms which keep living forms in shape, and are responsible for their building maintenance and repair.

Now the physicist's definition of a field is roughly this, when put into layman's language. When something happens in space as the result of something else happening somewhere else in space, and there is no visible means by which the cause produced the effect, the two events are connected by a field. The properties of fields are well established. They are stable and enduring. They can travel through time and space. They are indestructible except by the destruction of the causative object. The concept of a field is difficult for a layman to understand. Fields are invisible and intangible. They cannot be felt through the senses. Apart from the use of modern electronic instruments, they can only be detected by their effects.

Further research and experiment showed that the fields under consideration are by no means confined to the highly developed living forms such as men and trees. They are present in all living creatures, and indeed, in all living tissue.

For considerations of space I am jumping some ten pages to move on to Dr Pearce's comments on T-fields:

Some of the most impressive work in the field of thought transmission has come from Russia. As far back as 1921 the Soviets started to investigate the transmission of thought ... The man in charge of the investigation was Professor L Vassiliev, Professor of Physiology at the University of Leningrad. In a series of experiments carried out over a period of more than 40 years, Vassiliev showed conclusively that thought transmission does occur.

The most astonishing of Vassiliev's experiments centred around telepathic sleep suggestion ... Vassiliev was able to induce sleep in his subjects and to awaken them telepathically on countless occasions. Distance seemed to make no difference. On one occasion IF Tomashevsky, a physiologist, was able to induce sleep in a subject in Sebastopol, over a thousand miles away. Professor Vassiliev tried to screen out the telepathic waves by placing the receptor in a Faraday cage, and Tomashevsky, the sender, in a lead capsule. Far from screening out the telepathic energy waves, it seemed to work even better.

To this field – that is to say a field originating as a result of thought, which is able to produce effects at a distance where there is no visible means of connection between the point of origin and the point of effect – we may give the name of thought field, or T-field.

The importance of telepathy in the field of healing cannot be over-estimated. It probably lies at the root of all absent healing. Thought can reach right down to the body cells. Norman Cousins, the well-known American writer, relates in his fascinating book *Anatomy of Illness* how emotions of laughter and cheerfulness were able to produce a dramatic and permanent fall in his erythrocyte sedimentation rate.

Two Soviet doctors, S Serov and A Troskin, showed that the white cell counts in patients rose by 1,500 after positive emotion had been suggested non-telepathically and fell by 1,600 after the suggestion of negative emotion.

Psychic exponents of psychometry have been able to pick up information from inanimate objects, such as a ring, or a jewel, simply by holding the object in their hands, as if the T-fields of those associated with the object had become anchored in it.

Now minds are composed of memories and experience, and it is the amalgam of these which constitutes the personality. Most biologists believe that these are imprinted, like the patterns imprinted upon the tape of the recording machine, upon the substance of the brain. But bodies seem to be kept in shape by the body's own L-field, which is itself the amalgam of all the mini-fields of atoms, cells and organs. Can we apply the same concept to the mind, and say that each memory and experience is itself a field, and that in the same way as with the overall field of the body, it is the amalgam of these mini-fields of experience which constitutes the personality?

Man is a complex package of electro-magnetic life fields and thought fields associated with a physical structure of which the materials are constantly changing. This structure is maintained in shape and organisation by the electro-magnetic life fields, which are subject to the overriding control of the thought fields. Through the life fields he is an integral part of the much vaster fields of the cosmos, which are able to modify both the environment in which he exists, and, through that environment, the actual behaviour of his physical body.

Why so much space to L- and T-fields? Because they not only have a major part to play in the understanding of healing, but may well provide two firm stepping stones to prove the immortality of the soul. For those of you anxious to delve more deeply into the concepts of L- and T-fields, I refer you to *Design for Living*, by Edward Russell and *Blueprint for Immortality*, by Dr Harold Burr.

I would now like to refer you back to my example of Kirlian photography (see page 40). Here we have a practical example of field forces in action.

If we start collating these items we have some interesting data indeed. And it by no means ends there. I want to combine this information with the fact, yes the *fact*, of the aura.

Healing and the aura

In *From Seance to Science* (see page 156), George Meek states:

> English, German and American scientists have reported that on recent visits to the USSR they have personally witnessed colour moving picture films which show the human aura in great detail, reflecting changing thoughts and emotions. It is reported that Russian medical doctors now use this motion picture camera equipment for purposes of diagnosing physical and emotional illnesses.

Certainly several British healers use the aura for their healing work. The disadvantage is that you have to be a clairvoyant to be able to see the auras. Previously I have mentioned that Ena Twigg did this type of work, but the number of healers who have this ability is limited. One who does is Betty Shine who recounts her experiences in *Mind to Mind* (see page 154). I would advise any healer or would-be healer to obtain a copy of this book.

Centres of life force

When I studied yoga I was told of the *chakras*, centres of force, and perception. The normal teaching is that, as one progresses, so the *chakras* are activated. This is a progressive process and many mystics link this to the raising of the *kundalini*, energy depicted traditionally as a coiled serpent residing at the base of the spine. As this *kundalini* energy rises, so the *chakras* become more efficient as gatherers of universal life force, and spritual or psychic abilities are activated.

In the West we have tended to disregard this data, but I would like you to look at the two illustrations of the *chakra* points (see pages 118–9) and the way they relate to the endocrine glands, or ductless glands as they are sometimes called. My medical dictionary advises me that the endocrine glands, 'are a number of organs scattered throughout the body which secrete substances directly into the blood, instead of through a duct, and play a fundamental part in the control of growth, and intellectual and emotional development'. If we add

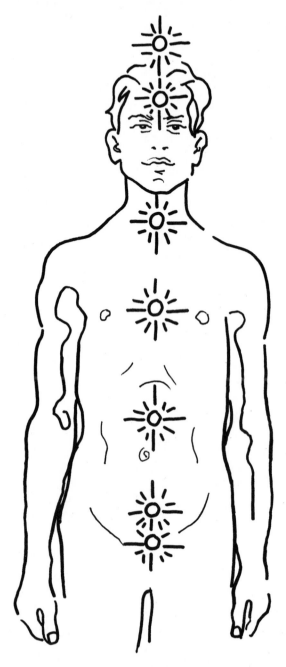

Figure 1. The seven chakras, energy centres which are associated with different levels of consciousness. Their relative positions are here seen from a frontal view. The chakras can channel healing energies.

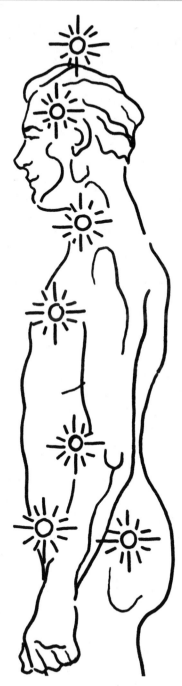

Figure 2. The chakra *centres and their relationship with the endocrine glands and main organs. Their relative positions are here seen from a side view.*

to the dictionary definition 'spiritual and psychic opening', then we may well be justified in using the terms *chakra* and endocrine gland as interchangeable expressions to denote points through which the body obtains external energy.

In *Stalking the Wild Pendulum*, Itzhak Bentov coined the term 'progressive sensory-motor cortex syndrome' to describe some of the effects that activating the *kundalini* can have. He is quite entitled to express himself in this way, being a biomedical engineer of no mean repute. Do not be put off by the term he uses; he has only done it to put the concept of *kundalini* into the terminology of Western physiology.

The point is that an increasing number of scientists are linking hitherto esoteric ideas with conventional Western pragmatism. At one point, not too far away, the various parts will be collated into a whole; my fervent hope is that whoever does it is capable of expressing ideas in a style which can be understood by lay people.

In practical terms I find that, when healing, I often concentrate on the *chakra*/endocrine points of the body. It seems that patients can best absorb healing at these centres.

Before leaving the subject of the *kundalini*, please let me give you a serious warning. Do not attempt to raise the *kundalini* by drugs or excessive meditation. To do so can be quite disturbing to you. There are people who say it is worth it; if you are one of these, be it on your own head. In my experience it is best to let things unfold as intended, not to try to speed the process up.

At the start of this chapter I said that nobody *knows* where healing comes from. But now you have enough information to draw your own conclusions, or at least, develop a theory or two.

Benjamin Franklin's Own Epitaph:

The body of B Franklin, printer, lies here like the cover of an old book, its contents torn out and stript of lettering and guilding, food for worms. But the work shall not be lost, for it will, as he believed, appear once more in a new and elegant edition, revised and corrected by the author.

Test your progress 8

The meditation I want you to undertake is for the gentle opening up of your psi perception, your parapsychological faculties. It is quite safe.

1 Sit in your normal position for meditation. Breathe slowly and deeply until you feel attuned.

2 When in this alpha state, think about the immense power of your mind. Build up this strength into a beam of thought.

3 Project this beam of thought to a place you know and of which you have fond and pleasant memories.

4 Let yourself travel back down the beam in time so that you are now there, not merely thinking of the place.

5 Enjoy what gave you pleasure, relive the experience.

6 Gently withdraw back from your journey to the present time, but keep with you the feeling of pleasure you enjoyed.

7 Come back to yourself in the normal way. Blink your eyelids, wriggle your toes and fingers.

This meditation and variants of it can be used to go back and perhaps forward in time; some claim to do this over more than one life.

9

Alternative and Complementary Therapies

To add further background to the healing process, the main
alternative and complementary therapies are described.
It is appreciated that there are many which have not been
included; reference can also be made to the titles listed on
pages 153–6.

As far as Europe is concerned, the EU may well introduce legislation of a restrictive nature which may inhibit both the practice of certain therapies and the sale of traditional remedies, which could even include herbs, food supplements and similar products.

In this respect the Institute for Complementary Medicine (ICM) is fighting hard to ensure that beneficial therapies and products of a non-toxic nature are still available to those who wish to use them.

As this book goes to press, the future of some complementary medicines is uncertain. Only by constant vigilance on the part of such bodies as the ICM and CHO can restrictions be averted. It is not enough, in the UK, to contact your Member of Parliament to let your views be known, you must also contact your Member of the European Parliament.

Acupuncture

This Chinese system can be traced back over 4,000 years.

The basic concept is that a balance must be maintained between *Yang* and *Yin*, the positive and negative forces in our body, so that the life force, *Ch'i*, can flow freely via the 12 meridian channels which, in turn, relate to organs of the body.

Along each meridian there are various points where needles can be inserted either to stimulate the system – for example to clear a blocked meridian channel – or to overcome pain. My comments are an oversimplification of a most complex system of healing. For example, a competent acupuncturist will test the 12 pulses in your wrists, six in each, which correspond to the 12 main meridians.

As in so many therapies, it is the therapist, not simply the method or system, which is all-important. The diagnostic skills have to be finely honed, with 1,000 acupuncture points to choose from.

It is essential that a fully qualified and experienced acupuncturist be consulted. The best choice of therapist is often found by personal recommendation.

Bach Flower Remedies

These remedies are obtained from the flowers of plants and trees that are picked under optimum conditions and then placed on the surface of pure water; after a few hours in sunlight, the flowers potentiate the water. The resultant stock is then mixed with a little brandy to preserve it. There are 38 Bach Flower Remedies, each treating a particular mood, state of mind or pattern of behaviour.

Dr Edward Bach, MB, BS, MRCS, LRCP, DRH, was a most distinguished medical man who was attracted to homoeopathy, and was pathologist and bacteriologist to the London Homoeopathic Hospital.

While accepting the homoeopathic concept of 'treating the patient not the disease', Dr Bach felt that the answer to many human conditions could be found in natural resources rather than drugs. In 1928 he started his field research and published his findings under the title *The Twelve Healers* in 1933 (see page 155). It is still in print; not many books are after 58 years!

Dr Bach's field researches continued until 1936, by which time a total of 38 flower remedies had been established. In addition a Rescue Remedy for emergency use was introduced.

I have used Bach Flower Remedies to good effect for many years. I always carry a bottle of the Rescue Remedy with me in the car, and have one handy at home. It is effective in cases of shock or trauma, or in conditions where stress may be experienced – say an examination or interview of importance. In a sense I use it as a non-medical tranquilliser. It has the advantage over a drug in that it seems to sharpen perception rather than dull the senses.

Full information may be obtained by sending a stamped addressed envelope, or overseas reply coupon if this applies, to: The Dr Edward Bach Centre, (for full details of UK address and telephone number, see page 149). There are official distribution centres in the USA, Germany, Australia, Holland and Denmark.

Do not dismiss the flower remedies lightly; the advocates include many doctors, among whom are Dr Charles K Elliot, MD, BCh, MFNom, MRCGP, MLCO, AFOM, RCP, Physician to Her Majesty Queen Elizabeth II, and Dr J Herbert Fill, MD, former New York City Commissioner of Mental Health. In a testimonial given in Gregory Vlamis's first-rate book, *Flowers to the Rescue* (see page 155), Dr Fill is quoted as saying, 'The Bach Flower Remedies are extremely sophisticated in their action. They are unusually gentle yet at the same time profoundly potent ... I use Bach Flower Remedies almost exclusively instead of tranquillisers and psychotropics, and I get excellent results. In many cases, they alleviate the problem when all else has failed!'

Chiropractic

People tend to confuse the work of chiropractors and osteopaths, who both utilise physical manipulation techniques. Chiropractors place greater reliance on X-rays and instrumentation to obtain an overall impression of the patient's condition.

In the UK, there are far more osteopaths than chiropractors, but as ever, the therapist rather than the therapy may well be the deciding factor when seeking help.

The initials 'DC' or 'NDC' after the name of the chiropractor denote membership of a professional body.

Herbal medicine

Herbs and plants have been used for the treatment of disorders in humans and animals probably since pre-history.

The owner of a health food shop may suggest treatments for minor complaints, but it is advisable to obtain professional advice before using herbs for a serious condition. It is one thing to use a herbal tea to counter indigestion, quite another to treat yourself with home brews unless you know what you are doing. Remember, many plants are poisonous. For example, belladonna (deadly nightshade) may well be of benefit in a homoeopathic tincture, but the alkaloid content when taken as a straight extract can kill you.

There are many excellent books on herbalism available, from Culpeper's classic reference work *The Complete Herbal,* published originally in 1653, to *A Modern Herbal,* by M Grieve, the most comprehensive guide I know, 913 pages, no less!

For everyday use my favourite book is *Herbs for Cooking and Healing* by Donald Law, PhD. For a list of these and other books on the subject, see page 155.

Homoeopathy

Samuel Hahnemann qualified as a doctor in 1779, but gradually became disenchanted with allopathic medicine. By the early 1800s, at about the age of 50, he had developed a system of medicine which, in quintessence, is 'treating like with like'. By that it is suggested that a medicine, which can produce an effect similar to the symptom of the disease, may, if administered in a minute dose, be efficacious in treating the disease itself. It does so by stimulating the body's natural defence mechanisms.

While there are many doctors in the UK who are homoeopaths, some practising through the NHS, there are also registered homoeopaths in private practice, and homoeopathic veterinary surgeons and pharmacists.

I stress that an holistic approach is taken by the practitioners, most of whom would maintain they are helping the body to heal itself. Indeed, Hahnemann stated that disease was caused by an imbalance of the vital life force, which he termed 'dynamis'.

The popularity of homoeopathy in the UK is due in no small part to royal patronage and, in recent times, the increasing search by many people for effective non-toxic alternatives to prescribed drugs and antibiotics.

Self-treatment by homoeopathic medicines is possible, but serious conditions require the attention of a qualified practitioner.

Biochemic remedies

Biochemistry is regarded by some as a development of homoeopathy, by others as a separate therapy. Certainly the basic principle is akin to that of homoeopathy, but the direction taken by Dr WH Schuessler, the founder of the system in the nineteenth century, was a rectification of the patient's condition by the use of tissue salts in homoeopathic doses.

There are 12 of these salts which may be used, either individually or in 18 combinations for given conditions. They are readily available from health shops and some pharmacies. The salts are normally self-administered, the patient looking up their disorder in *The Biochemic Handbook* (see page 155), or a similar publication.

I have used biochemic tissue salts myself and they certainly do work; many homoeopaths use the tissue salts in their practice.

Massage

There are few people who do not benefit from the loving touch of their partner or a close friend. Children too respond, even the 'Let Mummy rub it better' touch is, in itself, an important therapy. Gentle, soothing massage can be done by anyone and it is fine for taking the tension out of your shoulders after a long drive or hours spent banging away at a keyboard.

The real benefit of massage as a complementary therapy comes from treatment by a trained therapist. In cases of stress it is, I am quite sure, one of the best forms of non-medical treatment, depending as ever on the therapist. You feel pampered, soothed and cared for; in addition some aromatherapeutic oils are used in massage for specific conditions.

If a rapport is established between therapist and patient, massage often moves into the realm of healing. A skilled therapist is well aware of the meridian lines in the body and the *chakra* centres.

Naturopathy

The naturopath is trained as an holistic therapist. As I understand it, the basic concept is that Nature will heal, and indeed, if the body and mind are healthy, then disease will not get a look in.

To treat the patient, the naturopath will make a careful study of the background and medical history of the person being treated, and may well suggest a diet and, perhaps, a change of lifestyle. Any practical steps to aid recovery and a return to the natural norm will be suggested. To many, the naturopath's advice will seem to be 'just common sense', but the trouble is that common sense tends to be rather uncommon. In any case it is hard to be objective about one's own state of health, and a trained person can give an opinion on your condition which is quite unbiased.

There is nothing new about naturopathy. Hippocrates was an advocate of its methods, but you may consider it as a rediscovery or a 'green' response to the way many of us tend to live.

Cynics, while agreeing that many natural products and therapies are beneficial, point out that smallpox was overcome by the unnatural process of vaccination. Modern chemotherapy has wiped out some cancers that were once considered a death sentence. My own continued existence after three heart attacks is due to *both* allopathic and complementary therapy. The care I have had from understanding doctors combined with the benefits of healing from many associates has been, I am sure, a remarkable example of synergy.

This is not in any way decrying naturopathy, which is effective in many cases. I am, however, put in mind of the sage comments of the devout Arab, 'Trust in Allah, but tie the camel's leg'.

Osteopathy

An American, Dr Andrew Still, who was also a qualified engineer, evolved a system of manipulation which he called osteopathy. While many associate osteopathy with the treatment of a bad back or stiff shoulder, Dr Still's concept was holistic and not restricted to a particular area of immobility or pain.

The result of the way we have treated our bodies is studied by an osteopath when we go for a consultation, and if there is an obvious imbalance it will be pointed out. Often our occupation may involve undue strain on certain parts of the body which the osteopath may be able to rectify.

Do remember that a registered osteopath in the UK, recognised by the initials MRO and the title 'Registered Osteopath', has normally undergone a four-year full-time course of study at the British School of Osteopathy, or a similar establishment, and has passed comprehensive examinations.

There is no doubt in my mind that osteopaths develop a sensitivity of touch, not unlike that of some healers, which, combined with their extensive training, can give them an insight into what your trouble may be.

Under present UK legislation there is nothing to stop anyone calling themselves an osteopath. Having said that, I must admit that some of the old 'bone-setters', without a qualification worth mentioning, have the knack of putting things to rights if your back or shoulder is out. However, I must stress that if you go to an unqualified person you have to accept the risk that they may treat a condition which a registered osteopath or chiropractor might well refuse to undertake as a serious injury could result.

Hypnotherapy

The following monograph has been prepared by an experienced hypnotherapist, Colin J Page, Member of the American Hypnosis Association.

Hypnotherapy, like many other alternative or complementary fields of medicine, is finally gaining much wider recognition and acceptance as a valuable tool in the reshaping of our understanding and treatment of illness and disease.

The role of the mind in the cause or development of many physical illnesses, not merely obvious psychosomatic conditions, has only recently become appreciated more fully. This vindicates the necessity for an holistic approach to the treatment of medical conditions – both the body and mind must be considered in the healing process. Perhaps even more important is the need for such an approach in the field of preventative health care. Fortunately, we all possess extraordinary inner reserves of mind upon which we can draw, and it is to these very reserves, stored in our subconscious minds, that hypnosis can help us gain access and so harness them in the fight against disease.

There are many diverse areas to which these resources can be applied, and it is the function of the hypnotherapist to assist in this goal. Examples of such applications include: pain control; habit modification; treatment of anxiety, depression, fears and phobias, obsessions and compulsions, sleep disorders, stress, tension and related complaints. Unfortunately, however, there still remains a great deal of misconception, ignorance and fear surrounding hypnosis and its applications, creating blocks that can be extremely difficult to breach, blocks that prevent one from drawing on the immense potential that each of us has lying dormant within.

Hypnosis is a natural state of mind – an altered state of awareness – that is experienced by us all in many different forms, in different situations. And in none of these are we asleep, in the normal sense of the word. We are still awake, and aware of our surroundings, but differently so. Illustrations of these forms come in daydreams; meditative states; times when we find ourselves glued to the TV set or cinema screen, lost in a good book, captivated by an actor's performance, whether at the theatre or other venue such as a religious or political gathering, or sometimes experiencing blanks while motorway driving. In such instances the effect is to suspend temporarily normal critical reality, and facilitate an escape into a fantasy world, either to heighten an emotional experience, or allow a brief respite from the pain or boredom of reality. Herein lies the key to the hypnotic state; the mind is gaining something from entering this altered state of consciousness, and does so willingly. This negates one of the main misconceptions and fears of hypnosis, that a person loses control, relinquishing it to the hypnotist. All a hypnotherapist can do is guide the individual, to assist him or her to enter the state in a more structured way, and then direct the process towards the particular wishes and needs of that person. Hypnosis, therefore, is a consent state from induction to application, and requires complete trust in the hypnotist. Anything that may betray the trust will render hypnosis impossible. The notion of a Svengali-like demon wielding complete control over the poor, helpless victim is, to say the least, naive.

Throughout history, different cultures have taken advantage of this fascinating ability of the mind, albeit in apparently different forms. Older tribal groups employed trance states for ceremonial, spiritual or healing purposes, via the witchdoctor or his equivalent. Eastern civilisations developed various techniques of meditation (self-hypnosis) to similar ends. Here in the West it seems that formal hypnotic techniques appeared much later, although they undoubtedly existed in some form even in our oldest cultures. An early formalised state was propounded by Franz Anton Mesmer in the late eighteenth century – hence the word 'mesmerise' – and subsequently developed by pioneers like Dr James Braid under the term 'hypnosis' (from the Greek word *hupnos*, meaning sleep).

The modern-day professional hypnotherapist is trained in a wide range of applications, from medical to vocational or avocational, which can be grouped into three main areas:

1 Development of control by the mind over physiological processes.

2 Recognition and alleviation, via hypnoanalysis, of the hidden emotional basis of many problems.

3 Reversal of negative subconscious conditioning, and substitution with positive thinking.

There is an array of medical conditions that respond well to any combination of these treatments. Many of them may require all three, owing to the necessity for changes in both perception and subsequent behaviour. This is the world of stress and its insidious effects upon the mind and body over a long-term period.

Stress is inherent in our everyday lives. It comes from without and within. We cannot escape it: we could not function properly without a certain amount of its positive form. There are even those who are hooked on the adrenalin rush of such activities such as sports-car driving. However, problems arise when we are subjected to excessive stress, especially over a prolonged period of time.

When confronted with a stressful situation, the brain triggers our autonomic system to release adrenalin and other hormones. These prepare the body for 'fight or flight' and initiate a variety of physiological changes, all designed for self-preservation. This response is sudden and dramatic, and is outside our conscious control. It is an instinctive reaction to a life-or-death situation. When confined to such instances, this is a vitally important reflex action that subsides when the danger is past, with no harmful consequences. Things start to go wrong when, owing to the pressures of modern life, the stress response is triggered inappropriately by situations that are perceived as highly threatening, but of which our perception is distorted and exaggerated. This is the penalty for our developed consciousness, our unique self-awareness that is prey to negative thoughts and emotions. It is these aspects of our minds, both conscious and unconscious, that can gradually become a controlling factor in our responses, with disastrous results for our whole well-being. We can become imprisoned by our daily fears, insecurities, unrealistic expectations, unfulfilled desires, our ever-wayward ego, over which we seem increasingly to lose control.

As the high stress level becomes more and more chronic, we can succumb to a host of physical and emotional disturbances, often of a serious nature. Listed below are just some of these stress-related complaints:

Tension and migraine headaches	Skin complaints, e.g. psoriasis
Neck and shoulder pain	Anxiety
High blood pressure	Depression
Irregular heart rate	Insomnia
Asthma	Fears and phobias
Digestive disorders, ulcers	Stammering
Bowel disorders, e.g. irritable bowel syndrome	Sexual dysfunction
	Anorexia/bulimia
	Alcohol or drug dependence

The list is growing as we continue to discover that more and more diseases are linked directly or indirectly to stress, including many cases of heart disease and even cancer. Hans Selye, one of the foremost researchers into the effects of stress upon the body, has concluded that chronic stress levels can depress the body's immunological system, and hence open the door to any form of attack that would ordinarily be dealt with quickly and efficiently. We therefore need to strengthen our armoury in the fight against this hidden enemy.

As the stress responses emanate from the automatic, subconscious levels of the mind, the most effective means of counteracting them is by the use of those techniques that can gain speediest access to these deeper levels. This is precisely the area in which hypnosis is unsurpassed. As previously mentioned, the hypnotherapist can draw on several different approaches in the course of treatment. It may be sufficient to teach the patient how to harness the power of the subconscious in order to regain control over the physiological processes within the body. The mind, in hypnosis, is capable of exerting a surprising degree of influence over functions such as heart rate, respiration rate and blood flow, which are mostly outside our conscious control. It is these dramatic changes that enable hypnosis to be one of the deepest forms of relaxation for both mind and body that one can experience.

If the cause of the presenting condition lies in an emotional problem that has been repressed in the mind, hypnoanalysis can uncover such material and assist the individual to face and resolve the emotional pain. Age-regression is facilitated under hypnosis, which can be particularly beneficial if a person believes that current life problems may in some way be related to unresolved trauma from a past-life incarnation.

However, the cause is much more likely to be that we have simply learned to react stressfully in certain situations, leading to a negative conditioning of the subconscious. Eventually, we lose sight of the actual cause of the stress response; our perception of life and of ourselves becomes distorted; we are unable to maintain a balanced overall view, and are finally governed by these unseen destructive influences. Once again, with the aid of hypnotic suggestion and visualisation techniques, the hypnotherapist can help break this vicious circle by extinguishing the negative learned response, and substituting it with a more appropriate one of calmness and control.

Through this agency, we can provide some answers to a vast area of suffering to which few of us are immune, and as a safer, more natural alternative to potentially harmful drugs or even surgery. The ability of the mind to promote the body's self-healing process, as illustrated by Dr Carl Simonton's work in the field of cancer, is only just beginning to be seen more clearly. If we are to reduce this suffering in the future, the need to recognise and defend ourselves against those factors that negatively condition our minds is of paramount importance. This subconscious programming accounts for so many instances of inner conflict, frustration, low self-confidence and self-esteem, poor motivation and restricted accomplishment in all walks of life. Fortunately, we all possess the means to reverse the damage created and prevent its recurrence in the future.

New applications for the natural ability of mind we call hypnosis are continually being discovered, enabling us to draw further upon the vast untapped reserves within each of us. It is, however, ancient knowledge.

In conclusion

We have ranged from healing ourselves and others through to various alternative and complementary therapies and medicines. The treatment of a series of symptoms by a doctor is important. Without modern drugs, smallpox, typhus, syphilis, bubonic plague (the Black Death) and TB would still rage.

The trusted herbs of Culpeper worked in many cases, but as recently as 1901–10 life expectancy in the United Kingdom was only 45.5 years for men and 49 years for women. More recent data suggests that, by 1990–2, these figures had risen to 73.2 years for men and 78.8 years for women.

Of course, I appreciate that improved housing and nutrition have played their part – but so has medical science. And yet something else still benefits us outside the range of external treatments. The blending of medical science in all its forms with the healing arts of various therapies should combine to give us a synergetic panacea for the betterment of all. Idealistic, of course. But then, what is life without ideals?

Confederation of Healing Organisations Code of Conduct

The official code of conduct for the Confederation of Healing Organisations should provide useful reference to the principles on which effective groups can be structured.

Medical policy and ethics

1 Healing is legal in Great Britain. It is at present unregulated by law although it is increasingly likely to be the subject of regulations before long.

2 Government policy permits a doctor registered with the General Medical Council to use or prescribe healing (DHSS letter UNP/13 of 2 September 1985). 'Registered medical practitioner' is the description recognised in law for the individual usually called the 'doctor'. For the purposes of this Code the titles are interchangeable.

3 Successive presidents of the General Medical Council have said that a doctor is permitted to suggest or agree to a patient seeking help from a healer provided the doctor continues to give, and to remain responsible for, whatever medical treatment they consider necessary (GMC letter MRD/PW of 1 November 1977 and 6 March 1978).

4 *Patients' Rights*, the National Consumer Council Guide for NHS patients and doctors (published by HMSO), states under 'Alternative treatment within the NHS' page 17, that 'Patients in some NHS hospitals can request spiritual healing – providing the doctor treating the patient is told'

(Note: 1,500 hospitals agreed to this and it is believed that no hospital would in practice refuse such a request. Any instances of refusal should be reported to your Association.)

5   No NHS District Health Authority or Primary Care Division yet accepts healing as a therapy for which costs will be paid. Many local health authorities, PCDs, hospitals and hospital trusts co-operate by making a healing service known to doctors and patients.

6   The Royal College of Veterinary Surgeons accepts, as both legal and ethical, healing within the terms of this Code of Conduct.

7   The mission of the CHO and its members is to ensure that the role and importance of spiritual and lay healing is properly understood, to help healers to achieve the highest standards of competence and performance and to establish healing as a standard therapy on the NHS and in private medicine.

The Code of Conduct

8   This Code of Conduct is obligatory for healers belonging to members of the Confederation of Healing Organisations. It is, however, open to constituent bodies to have additional provisions, without in any way detracting from this Code.

9   Registered medical practitioners and members of other health care professions remain subject to the general ethical codes and disciplinary procedures of their respective professions.

10 The aim of healers within CHO membership is to offer to the medical profession and to the sick a service which is a complement, and not an alternative, to orthodox medicine. In particular healers must guard against the danger that a patient comes for healing for a known disorder without previously consulting a doctor and is subsequently found, too late, to be suffering from another serious disorder. To this end:

> a) A new patient must be asked what medical advice they have received. If they have seen no doctor, they must be

advised to do so. Since it is legal to refuse medical treatment no patient can be forced to consult a doctor. But the advice must be recorded for the healer's protection.

b) The healer must not countermand instructions or prescriptions given by a doctor.

c) The healer must not advise a particular course of medical treatment, such as to undergo an operation or to take specific drugs. It must be left to patients to make their own decisions in the light of medical advice.

d) A healer must never give a medical diagnosis to a patient in any circumstances. This is the responsibility of a registered medical practitioner. However, many healers have a gift of diagnosis, and in this case there is no objection to healers mentioning any condition or disorder which they may discover, provided they advise the patient to see the doctor for medical diagnosis and record this action.

e) Healers must strive for a good relationship and full co-operation with the medical authorities.

f) Healing must be given only in response to an invitation from the patient or their representative.

11 Guidance for healers visiting hospitals:

a) The hospital is responsible for the patient.

b) Healers must visit hospitals with discretion. In some circumstances distant or absent healing may be more appropriate.

c) If a visit is made to a hospital:

(i) Healers must not wear white coats. They may wear a lapel badge.

(ii) Healers must obtain permission from the senior nurse in charge before entering a ward and inform them of the patient's request for healing. In any case of doubt, the request must be obtained in writing.

(iii) When entry into the ward is obtained, healing must be carried out without fuss. It must be restricted to healing through the hands or quiet prayer.

(iv) If other patients request healing, the permission of the senior person in charge must first be obtained.

d) Healers must never undermine the patient's faith in the hospital treatment or regime.

e) If credentials are requested, healers must produce their association's current membership card, a church healer/visitor card, or other proof of membership.

12 Membership of an organisation forming part of the Confederation of Healing Organisations must be regarded as a guarantee to patients and the medical profession of the healer's integrity, sincerity and ability.

13 If the healer becomes aware that a patient may be suffering from a notifiable contagious or infectious disease, the patient must not be permitted to come into contact with other people, but be given a note to take to their doctor explaining the need for medical attention.

14 Healers are personally responsible for their actions. They must behave with courtesy, dignity, discretion and tact. Their attitude must be competent and sympathetic, hopeful and positive, thus encouraging an uplift in the patient's mental outlook and belief in a gradual progression towards wholeness.

15 Healers must disclaim an ability to cure but offer an attempt to heal in some measure. Recovery must never be promised.

16 Healers must not use titles or descriptions to give the impression of medical qualifications.

17 Healers must not ask for the removal of a patient's clothing except a coat and footwear.

18 When the healer is giving healing privately to a member of the opposite sex, it is advisable for the healer to request the presence of a third party whose bona fides the healer can accept.

19 Healers must never offer a clairvoyant reading during a healing session.

20 a) Healers should only heal in a conscious state of attunement. Trance conditions are neither recognised in law nor covered by CHO's insurance. Any individual concerned will be held personally responsible. If, for example, a patient suffers an injury while receiving manipulative treatment from an entranced healer it could result in a successful claim for damages against that healer.

b) Trance healing is forbidden for all research projects, when the healing is given as a service under arrangements with the NHS, and at public demonstrations.

c) Trance healing may be given to private patients who ask for it provided a responsible adult not in trance is present to safeguard both patient and healer. The presence of a third party does not absolve healers from full responsibility for their actions.

21 Healers sometimes say and do certain things while giving treatment because they are 'impressed' to do so. Reason and common sense should always be applied to such impressions.

22 To avoid offending some patients, healers must not raise the question of their religious beliefs unless this is invited by the patient.

23 Healers must not use manipulation or vigorous massage unless they possess an appropriate professional qualification. This does not preclude gentle massage or healing passes.

24 Healers should refrain from giving healing when they are themselves suffering from physical, mental or emotional stress.

25 Discretion must be used for the protection of the healer when carrying out private healing with patients who are mentally unstable, addicted to drugs or alcohol, or severely depressed or hallucinating. Such patients must be treated only by a healer with relevant experience who is accompanied by another healer.

26 Healers must treat as strictly confidential all information of a personal nature which is given by the patient.

27 Healers must keep adequate records for all patients and ensure they are kept confidential.

Healing and the law

28 It is essential that every healer, particularly any healer who practises a therapy outside healing as defined in this Code, understands and *observes* the law as it relates to healing practice. Disregard of the law may result in serious legal difficulties for the healer.

29 The law is enshrined in a series of Acts and Statutory Regulations principally associated with the medical and para-medical professions. In case of doubt, healers should state the facts to the secretary of their association and seek guidance.

30 In the light of legal provisions, great care is needed in the following cases:

a) A parent or guardian who fails to provide adequate medical aid for a child under the age of 16 commits a criminal offence. Healing is not medical aid as defined by the law, and a healer who treats a child whose parents refuse medical aid runs the risk of being considered as aiding and abetting that offence. Where it is known that the parents are *not* receiving medical attention for the child, healers are most strongly advised to secure the signature of the parent or guardian to the following statement:

'I have been warned by (name of healer) that according to law I should consult a doctor concerning the health of my child (name of child).'

Signed (parent or guardian) . . . . Date . . . .

Signed by witness . . . .

This statement should be kept with the healing records.

b) Do not practise dentistry.

c) Under the Venereal Diseases Act 1917 it is illegal to treat for reward, whether direct or indirect (e.g. for a 'contribution') syphilis, gonorrhoea or soft chancre. Therefore you may not give healing to patients suffering from these diseases unless the service is entirely free. It is legal to give healing to people with AIDS and congenital herpes. (Note: the British Medical Association say that provided cuts and sores are covered the risk from healing is minimal. The Department of Health say that in this situation the risk is nil. It is for the individual healer to decide whether to give healing to AIDS patients.)

d) Do not attend women in childbirth or within ten days thereafter.

e) The law relating to the sale and prescription of herbs is obscure.

(i) Do not sell herbs or herbal medicines without checking that this is legally permissible.

(ii) Do not prescribe herbs, herbal medicines or drugs unless qualified to do so.

f) The most likely risk run by a healer from a legal point of view is a claim in negligence for damages. It is essential that healers should make it quite clear that they are not doctors and do not purport to have the knowledge and skill of doctors. Healers must not treat a patient in any case which exceeds their capacity, but call in another healer or send the patient to a doctor.

Advertising

31 Healers may advertise that they offer a general healing service for all diseases, but they may not specify healing for any particular disease.

Animals

32 a) The Veterinary Surgeons Act 1966 prohibits anyone other than a qualified veterinary surgeon from treating animals, including diagnosis of ailments and the giving of advice based upon such diagnosis. However, the healing of animals by contact healing, by the laying-on of hands, by radionic instrument, distant healing by thought transference or prayer is legal and is acceptable to the Royal College of Veterinary Surgeons as both legal and ethical.

b) The rendering in an emergency of first aid to animals for the purpose of saving life or relieving pain is permissible. What constitutes an emergency must be a question for the judgement of the individual healer.

c) The Protection of Animals Act 1911 lays down as an obligation that if an animal clearly needs treatment from a veterinary surgeon, the owner must be advised to obtain this.

d) No breach of the Animals (Scientific Procedures) Act 1986 is permitted.

Insurance policy – contact or distant healing

33 All healers operating in the UK must be insured with the CHO Insurance Policy through the organisation to which they belong. This is as comprehensive as that normally used by doctors and permits the medical profession to prescribe healing or to co-operate with healers without incurring any liability for the alleged consequences of healing or of a healer's acts.

This policy only covers healers when they are carrying out spiritual or radionic healing in accordance with this Code of Conduct. It does not cover the practice of other therapies. The small premium also indicates that healing has no side effects.

Definition of healing

34 The Confederation has authorised the following definitions of healing for use by members:

a) For the purpose of the CHO generally, and of the Healing Research Project in particular, the following definition applies:

'Healing is the beneficial effect which healers in CHO terms are believed to have had on patients when, motivated by their own beliefs and following their normal practices, they administer healing in contact through the hands or at a distance by thought (or prayer) transference or by radionic instrument.'

b) For general use by members in relation to their own beliefs:

'A dictionary definition of healing is "to make well". To the extent that it occurs, healing is the transference of harmonising paraphysical energies. What energies are transferred depend upon the needs, beliefs, capabilities and procedures of the person or persons involved. Every living being is maintained by these energies which may be transferred in the presence of those concerned or at a distance.

'Healing may be of one individual by another; of a group by one person; of a group by a group; of one person by a group; or it may be self-induced.'

c) Each member of the Confederation is free to further define healing in their own terms in relation to their own beliefs without in any way detracting from this Code. These are outside the range of responsibility of the CHO.

Obtaining Help

The following section contains a list of useful organisations you may wish to contact. The names and addresses of organisations in the United States are listed separately (see pages 149–51).

Organisations in the United Kingdom

The majority of healers in the UK belong to healing organisations which are, in turn, members of the Confederation of Healing Organisations whose code of conduct is given earlier. There are two main groups in the CHO, the first of which is the British Alliance of Healing Associations. This, as the name implies, offers membership to associations rather than individuals. Thus for example, the Suffolk Healers Association will, in turn, belong to the BAHA. There is quite a high number of associations affiliated to the BAHA.

The BAHA runs national courses, as do the individual member groups. The BAHA also publishes a magazine, the *Alliance Review*. If you should require the services of a healer, the secretary of the BAHA will put you in touch with a local group if you enclose an sae for a reply. Their address is:

3 Sandy Lane, Gisleham, Lowestoft, Suffolk, NR33 8EQ.
Tel: not listed.

The second group, the National Federation of Spiritual Healers (NFSH), has a membership of individuals and not associations. This is the principal difference between the two organisations. The NFSH runs courses and also publishes a magazine, the *Healing Review*, which is also available to non-members by annual subscription. Members of the NFSH have their copy sent free of charge.

Requests for the address of a healer near you should be sent with an sae to:

The National Federation of Spiritual Healers, Old Manor Farm Studio, Church Street, Sunbury-on-Thames, TW16 6RG.
Tel: 01932 783164.

Both the BAHA and the NFSH have memberships in excess of 4,500 healers and probationers, while many healers are likely to have a direct membership of the NFSH as well as belonging to the BAHA.

The following groups are also members of the CHO. Please note, some of their telephone numbers are not listed.

The College of Healing,
Runnings Park, Croft Bank, West Malvern, WR14 4BP.
Tel: 01684 566450.

The Guild of Spiritualist Healers,
36 Newmarket, Otley, LS21 3AE.

The Maitreya School of Healing,
33 Shaftesbury Road, London, N19 4QW.

The Spiritualist Association of Great Britain,
33 Belgrave Square, London, SW1 8QB.
Tel: 0171 235 3351.

The Spiritualists National Union,
Stanstead Hall, Essex, CM24 8UD.
Tel: 01279 813636.

The World Federation of Healing,
2 Whitworth House, Buckhurst Road, Bexhill-on-Sea, TN40 1UA.

In addition to the CHO members there are other equally bona fide groups, including:

The Radionic Association,
10 Hurlingham Court, Ranelagh Gardens, London, SW6 3SH.

The Churches Council for Healing,
c/o St Marylebone Parish Church,
Marylebone Road, London, NW1 5LT.

The Quakers Fellowship of Healing,
Friends House, Euston Road, London, NW1.

The Harry Edwards Spiritual Healing Sanctuary,
Burrows Lea, Shere, Guildford, Surrey, GU5 9QG.
Tel: 01483 202054.

I am quite sure there are many other groups and healers who also do very good work, but are not affiliated to anyone. The fact that they are not listed does not mean they are not good healers. Mind you, to be even-handed, not every healer who belongs to a listed organisation may be the best to consult. The therapist, not the therapy, can be the deciding factor in who can bring you the maximum benefit.

The Homoeopathic Development Foundation maintains a good referral service for both information and treatment and can be contacted at:

19A Cavendish Square, London, W1M 9AD.

For Bach Flower Remedies and the address of the therapist nearest to you, write to:

The Dr Edward Bach Centre, Mount Vernon, Sotwell,
Wallingford, Oxfordshire, OX10 0PZ
Tel: 01491 834678.

A most excellent place of reference is:

The College of Psychic Studies, 16 Queensberry Place, London, SW7 2EB. Once again, do please remember to enclose an sae. Alternatively, telephone them on 0171 589 3292.

Healing organisations in the United States

Healing Touch International Inc.,
12477 W. Cedar Drive, Suite #202, Lakewood, Colorado 80228.
Tel: (303) 989-7982. Fax: (303) 985-9702.

The Association for Research and Enlightenment Inc. (ARE), 215 67th Street, Virginia Beach, Virginia 23451.
Tel: (757) 428-3588. Fax: (757) 422-6921.

Barbara Brennan School of Healing,
PO Box 2005, East Hampton, New York 11937.
Tel: (516) 329-0951. Fax: (516) 324-9745.

Healing Dimensions Foundation,
9462 Greco Garth, Columbia, Maryland.
Tel: (410) 740-4659. Fax: (410) 730-5265.

Acupuncture
American Association of Oriental Medicine,
433 Front Street, Catasauqua, Pennsylvania, 18032.
Tel: (610) 266-1433. Fax: (610) 264-2768.

Flower remedies
Flower Essence Society,
PO Box 459, Nevada City, California 95959.
Tel: (916) 265-9163. Fax: (916) 265-6467.

Flower Essence Pharmacy,
2007 NE 39th Avenue, Portland, Oregon 97212.
Tel: (503) 284-7090. Fax: (503) 284-7090.

Chiropractic
International Chiropractors Association,
1110 North Glebe Road, Suite 1000, Arlington, Virginia 22201.
Tel: (703) 528-5000. Fax: (703) 528-5023.

American Chiropractic Association,
1701 Clarendon Boulevard, Arlington, Virginia 22209.
Tel: (703) 276-8800. Fax: (703) 243-2593.

Herbal medicine
American Botanical Council,
PO Box 144345, Austin, Texas 78714-4345.
Tel: (512) 926-4900. Fax: (512) 926-2345.

The Herb Growing and Marketing Network,
PO Box 245, Silver Spring, Pennsylvania 17575-0245.
Tel: (717) 393-3295. Fax: (717) 393-9261.

Homoeopathy
National Center for Homoeopathy,
801 North Fairfax Street, Suite 306, Alexandria, Virginia 22314.
Tel: (703) 548-7790. Fax: (703) 548-7792.

Massage
Associated Bodywork and Massage Professionals,
28677 Buffalo Park Road, Evergreen, Colorado 80439-2267.
Tel: (303) 674-8478. Fax: (303) 674-0859.

American Massage Therapy Association,
820 Davis Street, Suite 100, Evanston, Illinois 60201.
Tel: (847) 864-0123. Fax: (847) 864-1178.

Naturopathy
The American Association of Naturopathic Physicians,
601 Valley #105, Seattle, Washington 98109.
Tel: (206) 298-0126. Fax: (206) 298-0129.

Osteopathy
American Academy of Osteopathy,
3500 DePauw Boulevard, Indianapolis, Indiana 46268.
Tel: (317) 879-1881. Fax: (317) 879-0563.

American Osteopathic Association,
142 East Ontario Street, Chicago, Illinois 60611.
Tel: (312) 202-8000. Fax: (312) 202-8206.

Hypnotherapy
National Guild of Hypnotists,
PO Box 308, Merrimack, New Hampshire 03054-0308.
Tel: (603) 429-9438. Fax: (603) 424-8066.

Alternative Medicine
National Institute of Health, Office of Alternative Medicine
(OAM), PO Box 8218, Silver Spring, Maryland 20907-8218.
Tel: (888) 644-6226. Fax: (888) 495-4957.

Further Reading

From the scores of books available, I have simply highlighted a limited number of titles which I have found helpful, both in my own studies and those of probationary healers whom I have been privileged to help.

In some cases I have added a few personal notes to give guidance as to content. It is a sad fact that many works are now out of print, but copies can often be obtained from shops which deal in out-of-print second-hand copies.

You will also find that most public libraries operate a special service whereby an out-of-print book can be obtained from the national library service for a small fee. Your local librarian will be of great help if you are not sure where to start looking.

The publisher or distributor may vary depending on whether or not you are in the UK. However, bookshops will be able to search their databases by title and author.

Healing

A Guide to Spirit Healing, Harry Edwards.

Harry Edwards, Ray Branch.
A well written biography by Edwards' own nominated successor.

A Guide to the Understanding and Practice of Spiritual Healing, Harry Edwards.
Develops and refines Edwards' ideas on spirit healing and may be considered as a suitable alternative to *A Guide to Spirit Healing*.

An Outline of Spiritual Healing, Gordon Turner.
For many years, the official handbook of the NFSH, now republished by the Psychic Press.

A Time to Heal, Gordon Turner.

This is the autobiography of Gordon Turner and if you read no other book on healing do, please, read this.

The Gate of Healing, Dr Ian Pearce.

President of the World Federation of Healing, the author was a practising GP, and he has included chapters on healing, stress and holistic and medical care along with a special section on cancer.

Mind to Mind, Betty Shine.

This is one of several books this author has written on healing.

Healing, Harmony and Health, Barney Camfield.

Laughing and Living, Barney Camfield.

Guidance not just on healing, perhaps more on life.

We Are All Healers, Sally Hammond.

An American reporter uses her skills to explore the world of healing and elicit the viewpoints of healers. Features Harry Edwards, Gordon Turner, Ronald Beesley, Christopher Woodward, Gilbert Anderson, Mary Rogers, Brigadier Firebrace and Lawrence Le Shan.

The Path of Healing, H K Challoner.

A study of in-depth healing.

The Healing Touch, H M Tester.

A first-rate work by an experienced healer.

The Origins and Properties of the Human Aura, Oscar Bagnell.

Psychic Discoveries Behind the Iron Curtain, Sheila Ostrander and Lynn Schroeder.

Beyond Illness, Dr Larry Dossey.

Professional Healing – My Way, Don Greenbank.

Design for Living, Edward Russell.

Blueprint for Immortality, Dr Harold Burr.

Alternative and Complementary Medicines and Therapies

Natural Health Handbook, Dr Anthony Campbell, MRCP, FF HOM.

A profusely illustrated large-format book which covers many subjects including acupuncture, herbalism, homoeopathy, naturopathy, nutrition and osteopathy.

The Alternative Dictionary of Symptoms and Cures, Dr Caroline Shreeve.

Over 500 pages listing the majority of common symptoms and diseases with attendant conventional and alternative treatments.

The Food Pharmacy, Jean Carper.

Over 360 pages in which the author demonstrates how certain foods can be of benefit in alleviating diseases and ailments.

The Practical Encyclopaedia of Natural Healing, Mark Bricklin.

Nearly 600 pages of advice on non-medical treatment for a variety of conditions.

Flowers to the Rescue, Gregory Vlamis.

An introduction to Bach Flower Remedies with information on Edward Bach and his work.

The Twelve Healers, Dr Edward Bach.

The Biochemic Handbook, Dr W H Schuessler.

Explanation and guide on how to use the Biochemic Tissue Salts.

The Complete Herbal, Culpeper.

Herbs for Cooking and Healing, Donald Law, PhD.

Includes outstanding colour plates of herbs.

A Modern Herbal, M Grieve.

This is really a modern version of Culpeper with over 900 pages. An absolute must for any serious student of herbal therapy.

Light of All Life, Dr Raynor Johnson.

One of the best works avaliable on karma and reincarnation.

From Newton to ESP, Lawrence Le Shan.
A work that covers the paranormal and healing.

From Seance to Science, George W Meek.
A well-illustrated book, bridging the paranormal and science.

The Reality of the Paranormal, A Ellison.
Large-format book in which readers can test and develop their own psi abilities.

Mind–Body Wellness, Jim Polidora, PhD.
A wonderful guide listing and commenting on books, organisations, journals, computer software and other resources.

Index